Atlas of
Pain Injection
Techniques

Commissioning Editor: Paul Fam
Project Manager: Cheryl Brant
Illustration Manager: Mick Ruddy
Design Manager: Andy Chapman
Illustrator: Jenni Millar

Atlas of Pain Injection Techniques

Therese O'Connor MB FFARCSI
Consultant Anesthetist, Pain Specialist
St Joseph's Private Hospital
Sligo, Ireland

Stephen Abram MD
Chair, Department of Anesthesiology
University of New Mexico School of Medicine
Albuquerque, USA

CHURCHILL
LIVINGSTONE

EDINBURGH LONDON NEW YORK OXFORD PHILADELPHIA ST LOUIS SYDNEY TORONTO 2003

CHURCHILL LIVINGSTONE
An imprint of Elsevier Science Limited

First published 2003

ISBN 0 443 06380 X

British Library Cataloguing in Publication Data
A catalogue record for this book is available from the British Library

Library of Congress Cataloging in Publication Data
A catalog record for this book is available from the Library of Congress

Notice
Medical knowledge is constantly changing. Standard safety precautions must be followed, but as new research and clinical experience broaden our knowledge, changes in treatment and drug therapy may become necessary or appropriate. Readers are advised to check the most current product information provided by the manufacturer of each drug to be administered to verify the recommended dose, the method and duration of administration, and contraindications. It is the responsibility of the practitioner, relying on experience and knowledge of the patient, to determine dosages and the best treatment for each individual patient. Neither the Publisher nor the author/editor/contributor *(delete as appropriate)* assumes any liability for any injury and/or damage to persons or property arising from this publication.

The Publisher

 your source for books, journals and multimedia in the health sciences

www.elsevierhealth.com

The publisher's policy is to use **paper manufactured from sustainable forests**

Printed in United Kingdom

CONTENTS

PREFACE

While the role of Anesthesiologists in the management of patients with severe or intractable pain has expanded dramatically in the past few decades, it has traditionally been anesthesiologists' ability to use regional anesthetic techniques both diagnostically and therapeutically that has made their contributions to pain medicine unique. This textbook emphasizes those regional anesthetic techniques that have been included in the Anesthesiologist's armamentarium for many years. In recent years, there have been dramatic advances in the technology of pain management interventions. These include implantable drug delivery devices, radiofrequency and cryoanalgesia neuroablation techniques, spinal cord and peripheral nerve stimulators, percutaneous nucleoplasty, annuloplasty and vertebroplasty devices. Despite these innovations, there is still a substantial role in acute, chronic and cancer pain management for many of the older, more conventional regional anesthetic techniques.

Nerve blocks play a variety of roles in the management of pain. For acute postoperative or post-traumatic pain, they may be continued throughout the most painful interval, serving as the sole analgesic technique or as adjunctive measures, reducing the need for opioids and other systemic analgesics. For patients with chronic or cancer pain, they may provide long-term benefit by reducing nociceptive inputs to sensitized regions of the spinal cord or brain. They provide periods of antinociception that facilitate physical therapy and reconditioning. Combined with corticosteroids, they reduce neural inflammation and produce neuronal membrane stabilization. They provide diagnostic information regarding sites and mechanisms of pain. Joint and muscular injections also provide an important contribution to the diagnosis and management of chronic pain. In the cancer patient, neurolytic procedures may provide extended periods of interruption of the most active sources of nociception. Long-term infusions of local anesthetics, often combined with opioids and other analgesic agents, can provide weeks to months of relief when systemic analgesics have failed.

Our aim in embarking on the preparation of this This text atlas was to provides a description of many of the basic regional anesthetic tools and the common joint and muscular injections that may be of benefit to patients with persistent or severe pain. It is unusual for these procedures to be curative on their own. Their value lies in their rational use in combination with other management techniques, including, but by no means limited to, physical therapy, exercise, psychotherapy, and systemic medication. All chapters in the book have been written to a template taking the reader through each block in a consistent and easy-to-follow way. Step-by-step illustrations accompanied by photographs are used to teach technique within the context of the surrounding anatomical structures and we have also highlighted where injections can go wrong and offered advice on how to avoid problems. It is our hope that this atlas will fulfill our aim of providing a strong foundation of regional anesthetic techniques in the treatment of pain.

Therese O'Connor
Stephen E. Abram
December 2002

Chapter 1

Mechanisms of pain transmission—an overview of anatomy and physiology

The term pain is used to define sensations that hurt or are unpleasant. There are however different types of pain. Pain following injury can be considered to have a useful protective function by rendering the injured area hypersensitive to external stimuli. Specific groups of primary sensory neurons carry stimuli defining the quality, duration and intensity of noxious stimuli from injured tissue. Their organized projections to the spinal chord or trigeminal nucleus mean that the origin of the stimuli can be precisely located. This somatic pain is often termed 'ouch' pain and is usually associated with acute, direct injury to tissue. It arises from structures that are innervated by somatic nerves, e.g. muscle, skin, synovium, and periosteum. Thus the pain is usually easily localized to the distribution of the nerve supplying the injured area, and is often sharp and intense.

On the other hand, pain arising from visceral organs is poorly localized. It may be appreciated as being deep in the body, often arising from the midline, or may be referred to distant structures. The reason for this is that visceral sympathetic afferents converge on the same dorsal horn neuron as do somatic nociceptive afferents, and both of these stimuli travel to the brain via the spinothalamic pathways. Thus, pain is appreciated in the cutaneous area corresponding to the dorsal horn neuron upon which the visceral afferents converge, accompanied by allodynia and hyperalgesia in this dermatome. As a result, reflex somatic motor activity may result in the spasm of muscles. Consequently, cutaneous nociceptors may be stimulated, which may be partly responsible for referred pain. In addition, there is considerable branching of peripheral visceral afferents with resulting overlap in the territory of individual dorsal roots. Compared with somatic nociceptor fibers, only a small number of visceral afferents converge on dorsal horn neurons. This overlap, combined with convergence of visceral afferents on the dorsal horn over

a wide number of segments, means that visceral pain is usually dull, vague, and very often poorly localized.

While damage to cutaneous or deep tissue is usually associated with inflammation of that tissue, neuropathic pain is significantly influenced by pathologic changes in peripheral nerve function. Thus neuropathic pain can persist long after the original injury has healed. Pathologic peripheral nerve changes include generation of spontaneous neural inputs, neuroma formation and regeneration of nerves. An injured nerve may become mechanically sensitive, and mild pressure or traction may produce bursts of rapid firing followed by many minutes of after-discharge, perceived as pain in the affected root. With time, the dorsal horn pain projection cells (wide dynamic range neurons) may attain lower thresholds and expanded receptive fields, adding to the traffic from pain fibers. The character of the pain varies and typically may be throbbing, shooting, lancinating, burning or freezing.

Recently, it has become apparent that the receptive-field properties of dorsal horn neurons are not fixed or hard-wired, but can change. The reason for this is that sensory input from primary sensory fibers and interneurons onto spinal neurons is normally too low in amplitude to generate an action-potential discharge in the postsynaptic cell. A temporal or spatial summation of postsynaptic action potentials is required to exceed the threshold of the cell. The center of the receptive field usually constitutes the firing zone, where an adequate stimulus will generate an action-potential discharge in the cell. Surrounding this firing zone is the subliminal zone, a peripheral stimulus evokes a response that is subthreshold. Changes may occur in the area because an increase in excitability of a neuron can convert a previously subthreshold input into a suprathreshold response, leading to receptive-field plasticity, or central sensitization. Thus, afferent barrages of high-frequency C fiber activity can generate changes in sensory processing in the spinal cord, leading to a hyperalgesic state. .

Careful investigation of the likely neurologic basis of each patient's pain may help in its treatment; thus whenever possible the following aspects should be determined: site(s), character, radiation, temporal pattern, factors increasing or decreasing pain, and associated factors. An attempt should be made to determine if the pain is somatic, visceral or neuropathic in origin, so that a rationale for treatment may be planned.

In addition, it should be remembered that there are other factors that determine an individual's level of pain perception. Psychologic factors are as important as sensory factors in determining pain perception and are more important in their contribution to suffering. Various responses to painful conditions exist, but depressive features tend to predominate in patients with chronic pain. Analysis of the patient from a psychologic perspective will provide a more thorough understanding of the patient's pain complaint and the ramifications thereof. Being attuned to psychologic issues will enable the physician to plan and execute a more comprehensive treatment plan. The relationship between depression, anxiety and pain is circular or reciprocal, rather than linear. The existence of pain often has detrimental effects on the patient's mood, increasing feelings of anxiety or depression. The development of depression or anxiety can exacerbate the experience of pain.

There have also been many reports about the perception and communication of pain, and its treatment may be influenced by sociodemographic factors. These include ethnicity and cultural background, as well as gender, age, education and socioeconomic class.

It is therefore important to approach the management of pain bearing foremost in the mind the varying influences on perception of pain.

On the other hand, repeated blockade of sympathetic activity with local anesthetic has been shown to reduce the severity of sympathetically maintained pain. Visceral pain may also be reduced by local anesthetic blockade of visceral afferent fibers that accompany the sympathetic efferents. However, the result is short-lived if pathology remains that will cause continued stimulation; for example, carcinoma of the head of the pancreas causes pain mediated through the celiac plexus. In these cases it is reasonable to consider neurolytic visceral afferent blockade for pain relief.

It has been demonstrated that locally applied corticosteroids prevent development of ectopic discharge and suppress ongoing discharge of injured nerves. Thus in the patient with chronic nerve pain, it is reasonable to consider injection of corticosteroid at the site of injury to a nerve, e.g. epidural or nerve root injection for nerve injury due to intervertebral disc pathology.

Degeneration and inflammation of joints can produce pain that is usually somatic in character, although this may sometimes be difficult to distinguish from neuropathic pain; for example, facet joint pain may be very similar to radicular pain. Joint arthropathy as a cause of pain can be confirmed by injection of local anesthetic into the joint. Addition of corticosteroid to the local anesthetic has been shown to decrease inflammation in the joint and thereby reduce pain.

The myofascial syndrome is a very common cause of somatic pain. It is associated with marked tenderness of discrete points (trigger points) within affected muscles, and with pain which is often referred to an area some distance away. In addition, the affected areas may have the appearance of tight ropy bands of muscle with associated autonomic changes such as vasoconstriction. Biopsies of such trigger points can show degenerative changes corresponding to the severity of pain (or can show little or no change at all). The most important aspect of the treatment of myofascial pain is to regain the length and elasticity of affected muscles. This is best achieved by physical maneuvers that stretch muscle. However, these maneuvers are often painful and may worsen muscle contraction. Therapy aimed at reducing pain and sensitivity in muscles is best instituted prior to stretching exercises. Trigger-point injections—injection of local anesthetic directly into the trigger point—can confirm the diagnosis of myofascial pain and a series of injections can markedly reduce muscle sensitivity. These injections, combined with stretching exercises, can produce significant analgesia for myofascial pain.

Transcutaneous electrical stimulation (TENS) applied directly to painful areas can produce analgesia during stimulation and often for some time afterwards. It is therefore reasonable to consider this non-interventional and safe method of pain relief for most types of pain.

2.1
LUMBAR FACET JOINT INJECTION

Anatomy

The zygapophyseal or facet joints (Figs 2.1.1, 2.1.2) are paired articular surfaces between the posterior aspects

Lumbar vertebra

Fig. 2.1.1a

Fig. 2.1.1b

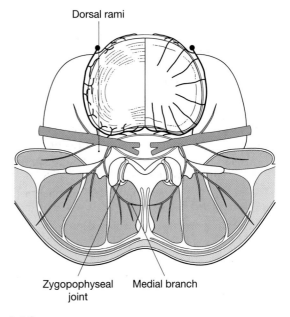

Fig. 2.1.2

of adjacent vertebrae. In the cervical region, rotation and flexion are possible as the joint surfaces lie midway between the coronal and the axial planes. Rotation is prevented in the lumbar region but flexion is possible as the anterior portion of the lumbar facet joints lie in the coronal plane and the posterior portions in the sagittal plane. In the thoracic region, the joints' inferior and superior articular surfaces overlap each other in an almost vertical incline.

The facet joints bear most of the shear forces when the spine is flexed. In addition, when the intervertebral discs are degenerated the facet joints carry increased load and weight, especially when the spine is extended. Innervation of the facet joints is via the medial branches of the dorsal rami of the spinal nerves. These nerves also innervate the muscles and ligaments surrounding the joints. Each medial branch divides into proximal and distal branches (Fig. 2.1.3). The proximal branch innervates the adjacent facet joint below, and the distal branch innervates the facet joint below. Thus, pain from irritation of a joint may cause secondary hyperactivity and spasm of the innervated muscles and may be difficult to localize.

The facet joints contain vascular, highly innervated intra-articular synovial inclusions, which may become trapped and inflamed when the joint is injured, causing pain.

Equipment

- 2 ml and 10 ml syringes
- 25 G needle
- 22 G spinal needle, end-opening
- Non-ionic radio-opaque contrast medium
- ECG, BP, and SpO$_2$ monitors
- Resuscitation equipment (see Appendix 4)
- C-arm fluoroscopy

Drugs

- Lidocaine (lignocaine) 1% 10 ml (or its equivalent)
- Corticosteroid if indicated, e.g. triamcinolone 25 mg (or its equivalent)
- Resuscitation drugs (see Appendix 4)

Position of patient

- Prone.

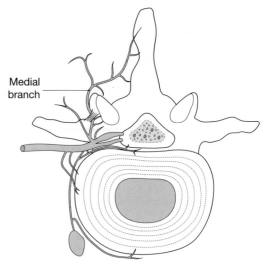

Medial branch

Fig. 2.1.3

- Pillow under anterior superior iliac spine to flatten the normal lumbar lordosis (Fig. 2.1.4).

Needle puncture and technique

- Intravenous access is inserted.
- Monitors are attached.
- Resuscitation equipment and drugs are checked and made ready for use.
- The lumbar midline and an area 10 cm × 5 cm laterally is cleaned with antiseptic solution.
- The spinous processes of the vertebrae are marked.

Fig. 2.1.4

- The insertion point of the needle lies 2–3 cm lateral to the cephalic end of the spinous process of the vertebra (Fig. 2.1.5).
- C-arm fluoroscopy is positioned at an angle of about 30°, tilted towards the side of the joint to be injected. The angle is adjusted until the joint is well visualized. A radio-opaque object, e.g. the tip of a hemostat is positioned over the joint and the skin is marked.
- Therefore, with the aid of fluoroscopy, the insertion point is identified.
- A skin wheal is raised and the area is infiltrated with lidocaine (lignocaine) 1%.
- A spinal needle is introduced in a vertical direction to the skin, until the needle is observed to enter the joint space (Figs 2.1.6 and 2.1.7). Confirmation of intra-articular placement is made by observation of the needle tip remaining on the joint line as the fluoroscope is rotated laterally (See fluoroscopic images of cervical facet joint injections on pg 18.)
- After negative aspiration, 0.5 ml of non-ionic radio-contrast medium (that is compatible with nerve tissue) is injected.
- The correct placement is indicated by outlining the joint with non-ionic radio-contrast medium, visible on anteroposterior and oblique views.
- When the correct placement of the needle is confirmed, lidocaine (lignocaine) 1% 0.5 ml plus corticosteroid, e.g. triamcinolone 25 mg, may be injected and the needle removed while clearing with lidocaine (lignocaine) 1% 1 ml.

Fig. 2.1.5

Fig. 2.1.6

Fig. 2.1.7

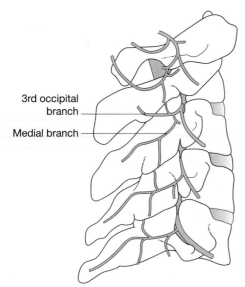

3rd occipital branch

Medial branch

Fig. 2.1.8

Fig. 2.1.9

Facet nerve injection may be carried out by placing a spinal needle at the point where the superior articular and transverse processes join as the median branch passes over the cephalad edge of the transverse process (Fig. 2.1.8, 2.1.9). Injection of lidocaine (lignocaine) 1% 0.5 ml plus triamcinolone 25 mg may be carried out for therapeutic effect. Diagnostic blockade may be unreliable as anesthesia of a facet joint means that both nerves supplying the joint should be blocked. However, this means that the joint above and the joint below will also be partially blocked and therefore diagnosis of pain in a particular joint using nerve block is not feasible.

Confirmation of a successful injection

- Relief of pain.

Tips

- Care must be taken to inject only a small amount of volume as described above. A total volume of more than 1 ml may damage the joint. If the joint is disrupted anteriorly, drug may spread to the epidural space.

Potential problems

- Solution may spread to the epidural space via the anteromedial capsule.
- Nerve root injection.

2.2
CERVICAL FACET JOINT INJECTION

Anatomy

The anatomy relevant to injection of the cervical facet joints is similar to that relevant to the lumbar facet joints. The cervical facet joints below the C2–3 level are innervated by the medial branches of the cervical posterior primary rami. These divide into lateral and medial branches after leaving the posterior spinal canal and the splenius capitis muscles cover the medial branch posteriorly. The medial branches lie in close proximity to the vertebral artery and the epidural space is in close proximity to the anterior joint capsule (Fig. 2.2.1). The C2–3 facet joint is innervated by the medial branch of the third occipital nerve which travels beneath the tendonous origin of the splenius capitis muscle where it may be accessed for local anesthetic blockade (Fig. 2.2.2).

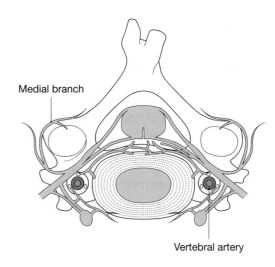

Fig. 2.2.1

Equipment

- 2 ml and 10 ml syringes
- 25 G needle
- 22 G spinal needle, end-opening
- Radio-opaque contrast medium
- ECG, BP, and SpO_2 monitors
- Resuscitation equipment (see Appendix 4)
- C-arm fluoroscopy

Drugs

- Lidocaine (lignocaine) 1%, 10 ml (or its equivalent)
- Corticosteroid if indicated, e.g. triamcinolone 25 mg (or its equivalent)
- Resuscitation drugs (see Appendix 4)

Position of patient

- Prone.
- Neck slightly flexed (Fig. 2.2.3).

Needle puncture and technique

Caution: injection of 0.5–1 ml of lidocaine (lignocaine) 1% into the vertebral artery may result in immediate convulsion and/or loss of consciousness with possible cardiovascular system (CVS) collapse.

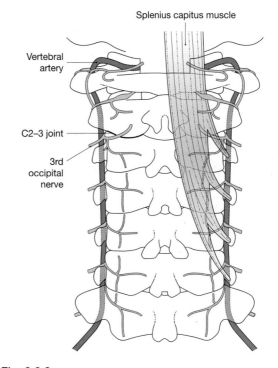

Fig. 2.2.2

- Intravenous access is inserted.
- Monitors are attached.
- Resuscitation equipment and drugs are checked and made ready for use.

Fig. 2.2.3

Fig. 2.2.4

Fig. 2.2.5

- The cervical midline and an area of 7 cm × 5 cm laterally is cleaned with antiseptic solution.
- The spinous processes are marked.
- The insertion point of the needle lies 2–3 cm lateral to the cephalic end of the spinous process of the vertebra (Fig. 2.2.4).
- C-arm fluoroscopy is positioned at an angle of about 30°, tilted towards the side of the joint to be injected. The angle is adjusted until the joint is well visualized.

A radio-opaque object, e.g. the tip of a hemostat, is positioned over the joint and the skin is marked.

- Therefore, with the aid of fluoroscopy, the insertion point is identified.
- A skin wheal is raised and the area is infiltrated with lidocaine (lignocaine) 1%.
- A spinal needle is introduced in a vertical direction to the skin, until the needle is observed to enter the joint space (Fig. 2.2.5). Confirmation of intra-articular

Fig. 2.2.6a   Fig. 2.2.6b

placement is made by observation of the needle tip remaining on the joint line as the fluoroscope is rotated (Fig. 2.2.6a,b).

- After negative aspiration, 0.5 ml of non-ionic radio-contrast medium (that is compatible with nerve tissue) is injected.

- The correct placement is indicated by outlining the joint with non-ionic radio-contrast medium, visible on anteroposterior and oblique views.

- When the correct placement of the needle is confirmed, lidocaine (lignocaine) 1% 0.5 ml plus corticosteroid, e.g. triamcinolone 25 mg, may be injected and the needle removed while clearing with lidocaine (lignocaine) 1% 1 ml.

Facet nerve injection may be carried out by placing a spinal needle at the point where the superior articular and transverse processes join as the median branch passes over the cephalad edge of the transverse process (Fig. 2.7). Injection of lidocaine (lignocaine) 1% 0.5 ml plus triamcinolone 25 mg may be carried out for therapeutic effect. Diagnostic blockade may be unreliable as anesthesia of a facet joint means that both nerves supplying the joint should be blocked. However,

this means that the joint above and the joint below will also be partially blocked and therefore diagnosis of pain in a particular joint using nerve block is not feasible.

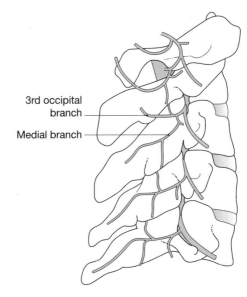

3rd occipital branch

Medial branch

Fig. 2.2.7

Confirmation of a successful injection

- Relief of pain.

Tips

- Care must be taken to inject only a small amount of volume as described above. A total volume of more than 1 ml may damage the joint. If the joint is disrupted anteriorly, a drug may spread to the epidural space.

Potential problems

- Solution may spread to the epidural space via the anteromedial capsule.
- Nerve root injection.
- Intra-arterial injection or intrathecal injection may result in immediate convulsion and/or loss of consciousness with possible CVS collapse.
- Hematoma may occur (avoid performing block on patients who have coagulopathy).

2.3
SACRO-ILIAC JOINT INJECTION

Anatomy

The surfaces of the sacrum and ilium form a synovial joint, the sacro-iliac joint. Ligaments and connective tissue surround the joint, conferring stability and preventing excessive movement of the joint (Figs 2.3.1 and 2.3.2). The joint is innervated by L4, L5, S1 (the superior gluteal nerve), S2 and L3. Localization of the pain is therefore difficult due to this wide nerve supply to the joint.

Equipment

- 2 ml and 10 ml syringes
- 25 G needle
- 22 G spinal needle, end-opening

- Radio-opaque contrast medium
- ECG, BP, and SpO_2 monitors
- Resuscitation equipment (see Appendix 4)
- C-arm fluoroscopy

Drugs

- Lidocaine (lignocaine) 1%, 10 ml (or its equivalent)
- Corticosteroid if indicated, e.g. triamcinolone 25 mg (or its equivalent)
- Resuscitation drugs (see Appendix 4)

Disaligned joint with pressure

Posterior sacro-iliac ligament

Sacrospinalis muscle

Fig. 2.3.1

Fig. 2.3.2

Fig. 2.3.3

Fig. 2.3.4

Fig. 2.3.5

Position of patient

■ Prone.

■ Pillow under anterior superior iliac spine to flatten the normal lumbar lordosis (Fig. 2.3.3).

Needle puncture and technique

■ Intravenous access is inserted.

■ Monitors are attached.

■ Resuscitation equipment and drugs are checked and made ready for use.

■ The lumbar midline and an area 10 cm × 5 cm laterally is cleaned with antiseptic solution.

■ The iliac crests are palpated and the intercrestal line is identified (this corresponds with the inferior aspect of the spinous process of L4 or may lie in the L4–5 interspace.

■ The posterior superior iliac spine is palpated with middle finger.

■ The forefinger is placed 4 cm above the posterior inferior iliac spine.

■ The insertion point of the needle lies just medial to the left forefinger and is marked.

■ C-arm fluoroscopy is angled toward the affected joint at an oblique angle. The X-ray beam is moved until the anterior and posterior joint lines are superimposed.

■ A skin wheal is raised and the area is infiltrated with lidocaine (lignocaine) 1%.

■ A 22 G spinal needle is introduced at 45° to the skin and advanced with fluoroscopic guidance, aiming for the lower 2–3 cm of the joint. A 'pop' may be experienced as the needle passes through thick fibrous ligaments and connective tissue.

■ The angle of the needle is then changed to 30° to the skin and the needle is advanced a further 1–2 cm (Figs 2.3.4, 2.3.5, 2.3.6).

■ After negative aspiration, non-ionic radio-opaque contrast medium 0.5–1 ml is injected.

■ The correct placement is indicated by outlining the joint with non-ionic radio-opaque contrast medium.

Fig. 2.3.6

- Lidocaine (lignocaine) 1% 1 ml may be injected for diagnosis of pain source.
- Lidocaine (lignocaine) 1% 1–2 ml plus corticosteroid, e.g. triamcinolone 25 mg, may be injected for therapeutic effect and the needle removed while clearing with lidocaine (lignocaine) 1% 1 ml.

Confirmation of a successful injection

- Reproduction of pain during injection and relief of pain following injection confirms correct placement.

- Radiologic assessment of the X-ray image post-injection of contrast may demonstrate tears in the joint capsule.

Tips

- While the joint may be easily entered, injection can be difficult where the joint is heavily invested with connective tissue and ligaments. This is especially true in elderly patients, where the joint is rigid and the joint space cannot expand to accommodate a volume of liquid. In such cases it may be possible to inject only as the needle is being removed from the joint.
- Sometimes, injection into the deep sacroiliac ligaments around the joint may be helpful for pain relief.
- Introduction of a spinal needle just above the midline of the upper sacrum and advanced at 45° to the skin, under the rim of the ilium and in the direction of the joint, will access these ligaments. Lidocaine (lignocaine) 1% 4 ml plus triamcinolone 25 mg may then be injected.

Potential problems

- Discomfort on injection.
- Epidural injection.
- Sacral nerve root blockade.
- Subperiosteal injection (painful in the awake patient).

Intervertebral disc disease may produce inflammation of spinal nerve roots, which may be the cause of radicular pain. The L5 and S1 nerve roots are most commonly affected, probably because they exit the bony canal through a narrow lateral bony recess, therefore increasing the likelihood of nerve compression and irritation. Lumbosacral radiculopathy consists of low-back pain that radiates a varying distance into the lower extremity, and which may be associated with motor and sensory loss consistent with damage to the affected nerve root. If bowel and bladder symptoms of dysfunction are present, large midline disc protrusion is suspected and prompt surgical intervention is indicated. Otherwise, if severe pain exists after treatment with immobilization and mild analgesics, epidural steroid injection may be carried out. Similarly, pain of thoracic or cervical disc origin may respond to epidural steroid injection.

Triamcinolone diacetate is the most commonly administered preparation and injection should be carried out as close to the affected nerve root as possible. Injection of a small amount of local anesthetic with the steroid will help to confirm drug placement and provide analgesia. In patients with S1 pathology the drug may not spread to the affected nerve root using the lumbar approach and the caudal approach to the epidural space may be required. Cervical epidural injection accesses the cervical spinal nerve roots, while in the thoracic region a paramedian approach is usually more successful.

3.1
LUMBAR EPIDURAL BLOCK

Anatomy

Structures encountered when inserting an epidural needle include skin, subcutaneous tissue, supraspinous ligament, interspinous ligament, ligamentum flavum (5–6 mm thick in the midline of the lumbar region, 3–5 mm thick in the midline of the thoracic region), prior to reaching the epidural space itself (Fig. 3.1.1). Beyond this space lies the dura mater, the arachnoid mater and intrathecal space containing the cerebrospinal fluid. The spinal cord usually ends at the L2 level (Fig. 3.1.2).

One should expect a distance of 3.5–6 cm from skin to the epidural space using a midline approach. In the lumbar region the spinous processes are generally perpendicular to the vertebral bodies (Fig. 3.1.3, 3.1.4). In the thoracic region the spinous processes lie at an angle of 30–45° to the thoracic vertebral body, thus making midline epidural injection a little more difficult, and sometimes necessitating a paravertebral approach.

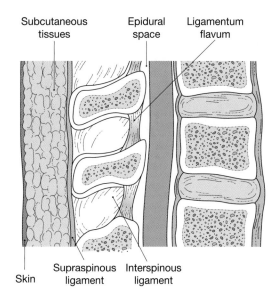

Subcutaneous tissues   Epidural space   Ligamentum flavum

Skin   Supraspinous ligament   Interspinous ligament

Fig. 3.1.1

Fig. 3.1.3

Fig. 3.1.2

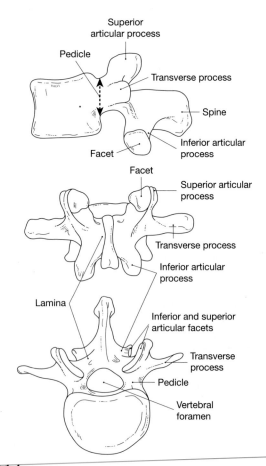

Fig. 3.1.4

Equipment

- 2 ml and 10 ml syringes
- 18 G, 20 G and 25 G needles
- ECG, BP, and SpO$_2$ monitors
- 18 G epidural set (Fig. 3.1.5)
- Filter aspiration needle
- Resuscitation equipment (see Appendix 4)
- Fluoroscopy (optional)

Drugs

- Lidocaine (lignocaine) 1%, 10 ml (or its equivalent)
- Corticosteroid if indicated e.g. triamcinolone diacetate 50 mg (or its equivalent)
- Saline (NaCl) 10 ml
- Resuscitation drugs (see Appendix 4)

Position of patient

- Lateral, usually lying on the side of the radiculopathy.
- Shoulders and buttocks parallel to the edge of the bed, perpendicular to the floor, with spine flexed.

Needle puncture and technique

- Intravenous access is inserted.
- Monitors are attached.
- Resuscitation equipment and drugs are checked and made ready for use.

- The midline and an area 10 cm × 5 cm laterally is cleaned with antiseptic solution and a fenestrated drape is placed over the sterile area.
- Lidocaine (lignocaine) 1% 2 ml is drawn up into 3 × 2 ml syringes.
- Lidocaine (lignocaine) 1% 2 ml, plus corticosteroid e.g. triamcinolone 50 mg is drawn up into the 10 ml syringe.
- NaCl 10 ml is drawn up into the 10 ml loss-of-resistance syringe.
- The iliac crest is palpated and the intercrestal line (this corresponds with the inferior aspect of the spinous process of L4 or may lie in the L4–5 interspace) is identified (Fig. 3.1.6).
- The spinous processes are palpated, and the level requiring injection is identified.
- This may be confirmed by fluoroscopy.

Fig. 3.1.5

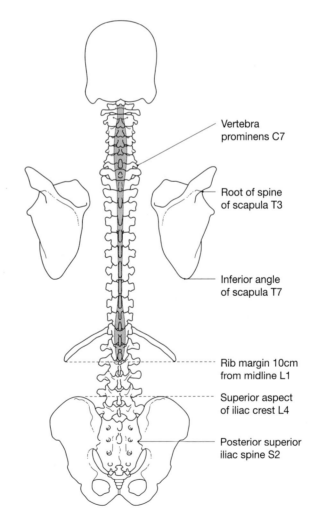

Vertebra prominens C7

Root of spine of scapula T3

Inferior angle of scapula T7

Rib margin 10cm from midline L1

Superior aspect of iliac crest L4

Posterior superior iliac spine S2

Fig. 3.1.6

MIDLINE APPROACH FOR THE RIGHT HANDED OPERATOR

With the left hand

- The fore- and middle fingers are placed each side of the interspace.
- These fingers are kept in place until the epidural needle is gripped by the interspinous ligament.

With the right hand

- The interspinous ligament is infiltrated with lidocaine (lignocaine) 1% 2 ml.
- The epidural needle is inserted, bevel facing the side of the radiculopathy, between the fore- and middle fingers of the left hand in a direction 60° cephalad, perpendicular to the spine, parallel to the floor, until it is gripped by the interspinous ligament (Fig. 3.1.7 a,b). In the case of thoracic epidural injection (midline approach), the point of entry of the needle should be as close as possible to the caudal end of the interspinous space and the needle directed 30–45° cephalad to enter between the spinous processes.
- The hub of the needle is gripped with the fore- and middle fingers of the left hand and this hand is steadied by leaning the wrist against the patient's back.

- The stylet is removed and the loss-of-resistance syringe is applied.
- The needle is slowly and carefully advanced, while constant pressure is applied to the plunger, the left hand aiding the advance, while at the same time applying a brake if required (Fig. 3.1.8 a,b,c).

a

b

c

Fig. 3.1.8a,b,c

a

b

Fig. 3.1.7a,b

Fig. 3.1.9

- At the point at which the needle enters the ligamentum flavum, absolute resistance to injection is experienced.
- At this point the needle is advanced very slowly until a sudden loss of resistance to the pressure on the plunger is experienced, the point at which the epidural space is entered.
- After negative aspiration for blood or cerebrospinal fluid (CSF), lidocaine (lignocaine) 1% 3 ml is injected.
- After 5 minutes the patient is questioned about any changes in sensation or power, and any changes in heart rate or blood pressure are noted.
- If the injection is for diagnostic purposes only, the needle may be removed at this point.
- If therapeutic effect is required, lidocaine (lignocaine) 1% 2 ml, plus corticosteroid if indicated, e.g. triamcinolone diacetate 50 mg (or its equivalent), may be injected. Alternatively, a catheter may be inserted through the needle if indicated (Fig. 3.1.9).
- The needle is flushed with NaCl 1 ml and removed.
- The patient is allowed to lie in the lateral position, on the side of the pain.
- Monitors should be left attached and i.v. access left in situ for at least 30 min.
- The patient is advised to contact the hospital should the anesthesia remain after several hours.

Confirmation of a successful block

- Relief of pain.
- Anesthesia in the distribution of the blocked nerves.
- For lumbar epidural steroid injection, improvement in straight-leg raising may be evident.

Tips

- Air may be used instead of NaCl to determine loss of resistance. If this technique is used it is advisable to avoid constant pressure on the plunger, as the air is compressible; instead it should be bounced intermittently with the thumb to test for resistance and loss of resistance.
- Advocates claim identification of CSF is easier with this technique.
- Advocates of the use of NaCl point out that absolute resistance to pressure identifies the ligamentum flavum, and that by applying constant pressure to the plunger one can identify loss of resistance earlier, thereby more easily avoiding the possibility of dural tap.
- An epidural catheter may be inserted through the needle and the needle removed, taking care not to withdraw the catheter when removing the needle. However, a test dose of lidocaine (lignocaine) 1% 4 ml with/without epinephrine (adrenaline) 1 : 200 000 is given after insertion, before any injection through the catheter is carried out.
- Injection of radio-opaque dye under direct fluoroscopy can confirm epidural placement.
- Insertion of a radio-opaque epidural catheter may be carried out also under fluoroscopy.

Potential problems

Immediate

- Failure to locate epidural space (sitting position may be successful).
- Intravascular injection (test dose important); addition of epinephrine (adrenaline) to test dose may help identification of intravascular injection.
- Intrathecal injection (test dose important).
- Hypotension due to sympathetic blockade (give i.v. fluid; consider ephedrine).
- Headache (possible dural puncture).
- Allergic reaction.

Later

- Infection (epidural abscess; bacterial meningitis).
- Aseptic meningitis; usually a result of intrathecal injection (test dose important).
- Cushingoid symptoms; usually as a result of repeated steroid injections.

3.2
THORACIC EPIDURAL BLOCK

Anatomy

In the thoracic region, the spinous processes lie at an angle of 30–45° to the thoracic vertebral body (Fig. 3.2.1 a,b, thus making midline epidural injection a little more difficult, and sometimes necessitating a paramedian approach (Fig. 3.2.2).

Equipment

- 2 ml and 10 ml syringes
- 18 G, 20 G and 25 G needles
- ECG, BP, and SpO_2 monitors
- 18 G epidural set
- Resuscitation equipment (see Appendix 4)
- Fluoroscopy (optional)

Drugs

- Lidocaine (lignocaine) 1%, 10 ml (or its equivalent)
- Corticosteroid if indicated e.g. triamcinolone diacetate 50 mg (or its equivalent)
- Saline (NaCl) 10 ml
- Resuscitation drugs (see Appendix 4)

Position of patient

- Lateral, usually lying on the side of the radiculopathy.
- Shoulders and buttocks parallel to the edge of the bed, perpendicular to the floor, with spine flexed.

Needle puncture and technique

- Intravenous access is inserted.
- Monitors are attached.
- Resuscitation equipment and drugs are checked and made ready for use .

a   b

Fig. 3.2.1a,b

a

Fig. 3.3.3a

With the right hand

- The interspinous ligament is infiltrated with lidocaine (lignocaine) 1% 2 ml.
- The epidural needle is inserted, bevel facing caudad, between the fore- and middle fingers of the left hand in a direction 60° cephalad, until it is gripped firmly by the interspinous ligament.
- The hub of the needle is gripped with the fore- and middle fingers of the left hand and this hand is steadied by leaning the wrist against the patient's spine.
- The stylet is removed.
- The hub of the epidural needle is filled with saline (Fig. 3.3.4) such that a 'hanging drop' appears (Fig. 3.3.5).

Fig. 3.3.4

b

Fig. 3.3.3b

Fig. 3.3.5

For the Right-handed Operator

With the left hand

- The fore- and middle fingers are placed each side of the interspace.
- These fingers are kept in place until the epidural needle is gripped by the interspinous ligament.

Fig. 3.3.6

With both hands

- The wings of the epidural needle are gripped with each hand, steadying the hands by resting the wrists against the posterior thoracic wall (Fig. 3.3.7).

Fig. 3.3.7

Fig. 3.3.8

- The needle is slowly and carefully advanced with both hands.
- It is prudent periodically to confirm high resistance of the needle in the ligament by testing with an air-filled syringe, then replace the stylet to make sure there is no tissue blocking the needle before resuming the 'hanging drop' technique.
- The 'hanging drop' at the hub of the needle is watched closely, and the patient is asked periodically about the presence of paresthesia.
- At the point at which the epidural needle enters the epidural space, the drop should appear to be sucked into the needle (Figs 3.3.6 and 3.3.8).
- After negative aspiration for blood or CSF, lidocaine (lignocaine) 1% 2 ml is injected.
- After 1–2 minutes the patient is questioned about changes in sensation or power, and any changes in heart rate or blood pressure are noted.
- If the injection is for diagnostic purposes only, the needle may be removed at this point.
- If therapeutic effect is required, lidocaine (lignocaine) 1% 1 ml plus corticosteroid, e.g. triamcinolone 50 mg, may be injected.
- The patient is allowed to lie in the lateral position, on the side of the pain.
- Monitors should be left attached and i.v. access kept in situ for at least 30 min.

Confirmation of a successful block

- Relief of pain

Tips

- Loss-of-resistance techniques may also be used to access the cervical epidural space.
- The steroid may be given soon after the test dose, as hypotension may be a problem if the patient remains in the sitting position.

Potential problems

Immediate

- Failure to locate epidural space (lateral position with loss of resistance technique may be successful).
- Pain on injection (caution: close proximity to spinal cord).
- Intrathecal injection (test dose important).

- Hypotension +/– bradycardia due to sympathetic blockade (maximum 3 ml local anesthetic administered in this technique).
- Vasovagal syncope is common in young adult patients.
- Intravascular injection; addition of epinephrine (adrenaline) 1 : 200 000 to the test dose may aid identification of intravascular injection.
- Headache (possible dural puncture).
- Allergic reaction.

- Spinal cord injury may occur if the epidural space is not recognized. Deep sedation should be avoided during needle insertion and drug injection.

Later

- Infection (epidural abscess, bacterial meningitis).
- Aseptic meningitis, usually the result of intrathecal injection (test dose important).
- Cushingoid symptoms (usually as a result of repeated injections).

3.4
CAUDAL EPIDURAL BLOCK

Anatomy

Injection of anesthetic through the sacral hiatus allows access to the sacral epidural space or caudal anesthesia. The sacrum is roughly triangular in shape and is made up of five fused sacral vertebrae (Fig. 3.4.1). Its dorsal aspect is convex and there is a midline sacral canal that allows passage through four pairs of foramen, anteriorly and posteriorly, of the sacral nerves. At the caudal end lies the coccyx, and at the cephalad end lies the fifth lumbar vertebra. The posterior wall of S5, and sometimes S4, is unfused. The thick fibrous sacrococcygeal membrane or sacral hiatus covers the defect. This may be variable in size as the posterior wall of other sacral vertebrae may also be unfused. Penetration of this membrane allows access to the sacral epidural space.

Equipment

- 2 ml, 5 ml and 20 ml syringes
- 18 G, 20 G and 25 G needle
- 22 G, 3–5 cm short-bevel needle, with stylet
- ECG, BP, and SpO$_2$ monitors
- Resuscitation equipment (see Appendix 4)
- Fluoroscopy (optional)

Drugs

- Lidocaine (lignocaine) 1%, 10 ml (or its equivalent)

- Corticosteroid if indicated, e.g. triamcinolone diacetate 50 mg (or its equivalent)
- Saline (NaCl) 10 ml
- Resuscitation drugs (see Appendix 4)

Position of patient

- Prone.
- Pillow under abdomen and/or operating table broken to allow flexion of the lumbo-sacral spine (Fig. 3.4.2).

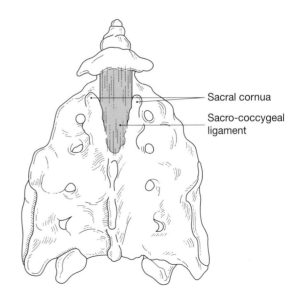

Sacral cornua

Sacro-coccygeal ligament

Fig. 3.4.1

- Lower limbs abducted 15°, toes rotated to point towards the opposite foot (Fig. 3.4.3).

Needle puncture and technique (adult)

- Intravenous access is inserted.
- Monitors are attached.
- Resuscitation equipment and drugs are checked and made ready for use.

Fig. 3.4.2

Fig. 3.4.3

- The midline and an area 10 cm × 5 cm laterally is cleaned with antiseptic solution with antiseptic solution and a fenestrated drape is placed over the sterile area.
- Lidocaine (lignocaine) 1% 2 ml is drawn up into three 2 ml syringes.
- Lidocaine (lignocaine) 1% 15 ml plus corticosteroid, e.g. triamcinolone 50 mg, is drawn up into the 20 ml syringe.
- NaCl 10 ml is drawn up into the 10 ml syringe.

For the Right-handed Operator

With the left hand

- The posterior superior iliac spines are identified.
- The sacral cornua (the unfused spinous processes of S5) are also identified and marked.
- Between the cornua lies the base of the sacral hiatus, a roughly triangular fibroelastic structure.
- The index and middle fingers of the left hand are placed on each of the sacral cornua (Fig. 3.4.4).
- The insertion point lies between these two fingers.

With the right hand

- The insertion point is infiltrated with lidocaine (lignocaine) 1% 2 ml.
- The 22 G short-bevel needle with stylet is inserted at an angle of 45° to the skin.

Sacral cornua

Fig. 3.4.4

Fig. 4.1.5

Fig. 4.1.7

Fig. 4.1.6

Fig. 4.1.8

hand in a direction 15–20° cephalad, until it makes contact with the rib (Figs 4.1.6 and 4.1.7).

- The needle-hub is gripped with the fingers of the left hand and this hand is steadied by leaning the wrist against the patient's posterior chest wall (Fig. 4.1.8).

- With the right and left hands acting as one unit the needle is walked off the edge of the rib until it enters the intercostal space immediately below the rib (Fig. 4.1.9).

- It is then advanced 2 mm.

- After negative aspiration, 3–4 ml of local anesthetic, plus corticosteroid if indicated, is injected (Fig. 4.1.10) and the needle is withdrawn.

- Monitors are left attached and i.v. access left in situ for at least 30 min.

- Chest X-ray is performed if pneumothorax is suspected.

Fig. 4.1.9

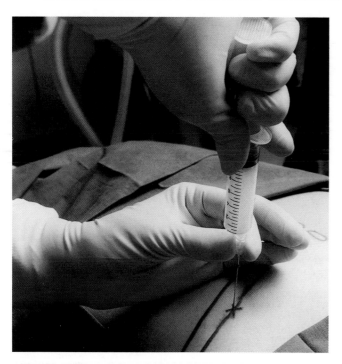

Fig. 4.1.10

Confirmation of a successful block

■ Relief of pain.
■ Anesthesia in the distribution of the blocked nerve.

Tips

■ The approximate depth to the rib may be determined with the left fore- and middle fingers before insertion of the needle.

■ Insertion of the needle > 2 mm deeper than the rib when intercostal space is reached is avoided. This will minimize the risk of pneumothorax, as the average distance from the rib to the pleura is 8 mm. If patient coughs on injection, pneumothorax is suspected.

■ Doppler ultrasound can aid performance of this block by identifying the neurovascular bundle.

■ Neurolytic intercostal nerve block, e.g. with alcohol 50% 3 ml (made up by combining equal parts of alcohol 100% and lidocaine (lignocaine) 1% or its equivalent), or phenol 6%, may be carried out after local anesthetic block confirms accurate placement of the needle as described above. However, it is important to note that injection may result in subarachnoid spread of a neurolytic agent. Injection of non-ionic radio-constrast medium may aid accurate placement of needle in neurolytic block (Fig. 4.1.11).

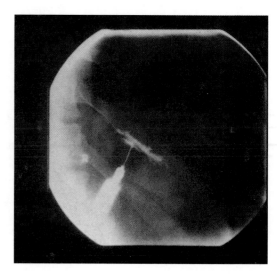

Fig. 4.1.11

■ Placement of a catheter into the intercostal space can be achieved by threading 3 cm of catheter through an 18 G epidural needle after the intercostal neurovascular bundle has been identified as above.

Potential problems

■ Injection within the nerve sheath can result in the spread of anesthetic to the subarachnoid space.

■ Intercostal block in patients with severe respiratory problems should be avoided as there is risk of a pneumothorax. Careful observation of a small pneumothorax is usually all that is required but failure to re-expand the lung may require chest tube insertion.

■ Because of the vascularity of the intercostal space, there may be rapid absorption of local anesthetic and systemic effects can occur quickly, especially with multiple blocks. However, peak plasma concentration of local anesthetic may occur 15–20 minutes after the block is performed, when systemic toxicity effects may develop. Addition of epinephrine (adrenaline) to the anesthetic solution may decrease the peak plasma concentration of local anesthetic.

■ If aspiration of blood occurs, the needle should be removed, keeping the left fore- and middle fingers in place. The needle is cleared, reinserted to contact the rib again, and the block is continued as above.

■ Care of the airway must be remembered if sedation is administered to a patient in the prone position.

4.2
INTERPLEURAL BLOCK

Anatomy

The parietal pleura lines the thoracic wall, the thoracic surface of the diaphragm and the lateral mediastinum. The visceral pleura completely covers the surface of the lung. Both the pleural layers become contiguous at the root of the lung. Between the two pleural layers lies the interpleural space (Fig. 4.2.1). Injection of local anesthetic into this space produces an interpleural block by topical contact with free nerve endings within the pleura, and by local diffusion to nerves in the vicinity of injection. These include the intercostal nerves, the sympathetic chain, and the inferior part of the brachial plexus. Local anesthetic solution may also track to the epidural and subarachnoid spaces producing blockade.

Equipment

- 2 ml and 10 ml syringes
- 18 G, 20 G and 25 G needles
- ECG, BP, and SpO$_2$ monitors
- 18 G epidural set
- Well-lubricated 5 ml glass syringe
- Resuscitation equipment (see Appendix 4)

Drugs

- Lidocaine (lignocaine) 1% 10 ml
- Levobupivacaine 0.25%, 20 ml (or its equivalent)
- Saline (NaCl) 10 ml
- Resuscitation drugs (see Appendix 4)

Position of patient

The technique described here relies on negative interpleural pressure to identify the interpleural space. Therefore the patient should be breathing spontaneously for this technique.

- Semi-prone
- Side to be blocked uppermost, supported by a pillow (Fig. 4.2.2).
- The arm should be allowed to fall forwards in front of the body to rotate the scapula anterolaterally.

Interpleural space

Fig. 4.2.1

Fig. 4.2.2

Needle puncture and technique

- Intravenous access is inserted.
- Monitors are attached.
- Resuscitation equipment and drugs are checked and made ready for use.
- The midline and an area 15 cm × 12 cm laterally is cleaned with antiseptic solution and a fenestrated drape is placed over the sterile area.
- Lidocaine (lignocaine) 2%, 2 ml is drawn up.
- Levobupivicaine 0.25% 20 ml is drawn up.
- Air is drawn up into a well-lubricated 5 ml syringe.
- The seventh and eighth ribs are palpated and marked.
- A point approximately 10 cm from the midline, immediately *superior* to the eighth rib is marked; this is the insertion point (Fig. 4.2.3).

For the Right-handed Operator

With the left hand

- The fore- and middle fingers are placed each side of the insertion point, palpating the superior aspect of the eighth rib.
- These fingers are kept in place until the epidural needle passes through the subcutaneous tissue.

With the right hand

- A skin wheal is raised at the insertion point.
- The epidural needle is inserted between the fore- and middle fingers of the left hand, taking care that the point of entry of the needle is as close as possible to the superior aspect of the eighth rib. This helps to avoid damage to the neurovascular bundle, which lies immediately inferior to the seventh rib.
- After passage through the subcutaneous tissue, the hub of the needle is gripped with the fore- and middle fingers of the left hand and this hand is steadied by leaning the wrist against the patient's posterior chest wall.
- The stylet is removed and the well-lubricated glass syringe containing 3 ml air is applied (Fig. 4.2.4).
- The needle is slowly and carefully advanced, with no pressure applied to the plunger, the left hand aiding the advance, while at the same time applying a brake if required.
- Resistance from the tissues prevents the plunger from advancing.
- At the point at which the needle enters the interpleural space a definite click is experienced, negative pressure draws the air in and the barrel drops (Fig. 4.2.5 a,b).

Fig. 4.2.3

Fig. 4.2.4

Fig. 4.3.2

a

Fig. 4.3.3a

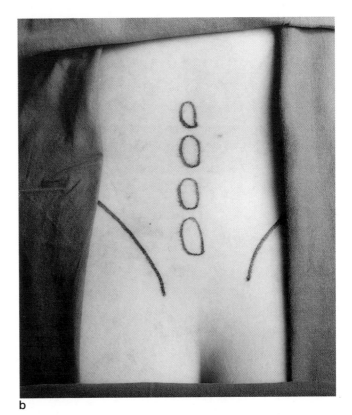

b

Fig. 4.3.3b

The nerve corresponding to each vertebra emerges just below the transverse process of that vertebra at this site (see Appendix 6).

■ Therefore, with the aid of fluoroscopy, the insertion point is identified.

■ A skin wheal is raised and the area is infiltrated with lidocaine (lignocaine) 1%.

■ A spinal needle is introduced in a vertical direction to the skin, until the needle contacts bone at an approximate depth of 3–5 cm, the transverse process of that vertebra (Fig. 4.3.4 a,b,c).

a

b

c

Fig. 4.3.4a,b,c

- The needle is then walked off the transverse process in the caudad direction and advanced 1.5–2 cm, the site of the emerging nerve root (Fig. 4.3.5).
- It is useful to confirm the needle tip over the intervertebral foramen with fluoroscopy.
- Paresthesia in the distribution of the nerve may be experienced.
- After aspiration, non-ionic radio-opaque contrast medium 1 ml is injected (Fig. 4.3.6).
- The correct placement is indicated by outlining the nerve root with non-ionic radio-opaque contrast medium, visible on anteroposterior and lateral fluoroscopic views (Fig. 4.3.7; note that this shows L3 not L5).
- After further aspiration, lidocaine (lignocaine) 1% 0.5–1 ml is injected.
- After 5 minutes the patient is questioned about changes in pain, sensation and power of the lower limb.
- For diagnostic nerve root blockade, the needle may be removed when the level causing pain is identified.
- Alternatively, when the level is identified lidocaine (lignocaine) 1% 1 ml plus corticosteroid, e.g. triamcinolone 25 mg may be injected for therapeutic effect and the needle removed while clearing with local anesthetic.

Fig. 4.3.6

Sympathetic chain   Lumbar nerve

Fig. 4.3.5

Fig. 4.3.7

Confirmation of a successful block

- Relief of pain and anesthesia in distribution of the blocked nerve.

Tips

- As in the case of thoracic nerve root block, it has also been recommended that the needle is angled 20° medially after entering the paravertebral space. However care must be taken, with the aid of fluoroscopy, not to inject local anesthetic solution into the nerve sheath allowing tracking of the solution centrally to produce intrathecal blockade.

Potential problems

- Intrathecal injection.
- Epidural blockade usually occurs with this block, but this is not a problem once low volumes are used. However, even small volumes of epidural spread may confound the diagnostic value of the block.
- Sympathetic blockade is unlikely, but it may occur and cause hemodynamic changes.

4.4
THORACIC NERVE ROOT BLOCK

Anatomy

The anatomy relevant to thoracic paravertebral nerve root blockade is very similar to the anatomy relevant to lumbar paravertebral nerve root block, except that:

■ ribs are present instead of the rudimentary ribs of the lumbar spine, the transverse processes;

■ the lung and pleura are in close proximity to the injection site, therefore the risk of pneumothorax is significant;

■ unlike the lumbar region, where the needle passes through the substance of the psoas muscle, the needle passes through connective tissue only in the thoracic region (Fig. 4.4.1 a,b,c);

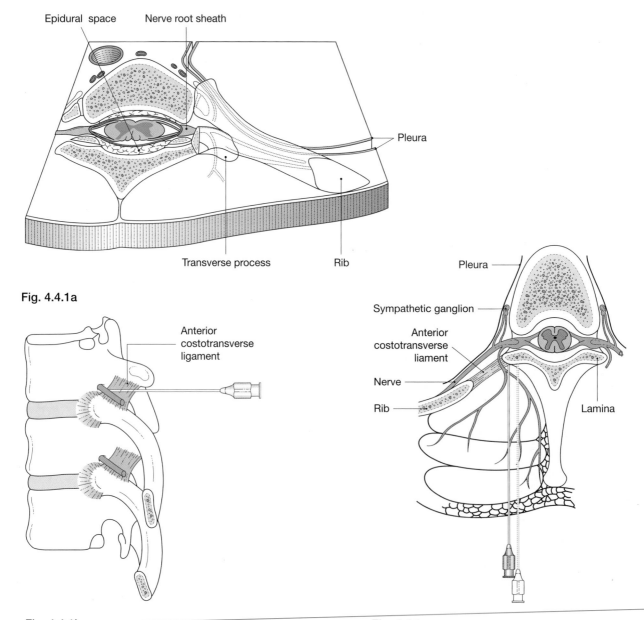

Epidural space

Nerve root sheath

Pleura

Transverse process

Rib

Fig. 4.4.1a

Anterior costotransverse ligament

Fig. 4.4.1b

Pleura

Sympathetic ganglion

Anterior costotransverse liament

Nerve

Rib

Lamina

Fig. 4.4.1c

usually the anterior opening of the foramen that is the most prominent.

■ The insertion point of the needle lies 2–3 cm lateral to the midline (variable) and approximately 1 cm medial to the posterior iliac spine (Figs 4.5.4, 4.5.5).

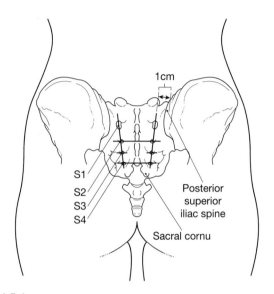

Fig. 4.5.4

■ Therefore, with the aid of fluoroscopy, the insertion point is identified.

■ A skin wheal is raised and the area is infiltrated with lidocaine (lignocaine) 1%.

■ A spinal needle is introduced in a vertical direction to the skin, and aimed slightly cephalad until bone is contacted (Fig. 4.5.6).

■ The needle is then walked off the sacrum in a caudad direction until it slips into the foramen. After confirmation with the aid of fluoroscopy it is then advanced 1 cm.

■ Paresthesia may be produced.

■ After aspiration, non-ionic radio-opaque contrast medium 1 ml is injected (Fig. 4.5.7).

■ The correct placement is indicated by a needle tip flush with the anterior surface of the sacrum.

■ After further aspiration, lidocaine (lignocaine) 1% 0.5 ml is injected.

■ After 5 min, the patient is questioned about changes in pain, sensation and power of the lower limb.

■ For diagnostic nerve root blockade the needle may be removed when the level causing pain is identified.

Fig. 4.5.5

Fig. 4.5.6

Fig. 4.5.7

Fig. 4.5.9

Fig. 4.5.8

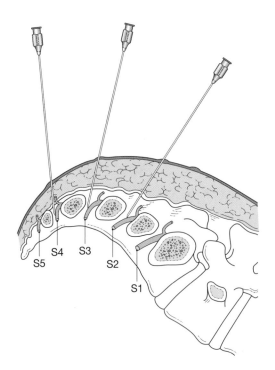

Fig. 4.5.10

■ Alternatively, when the level is identified, lidocaine (lignocaine) 1% 1 ml plus corticosteroid, e.g. triamcinolone 25 mg, may be injected for therapeutic effect and the needle removed while clearing needle with local anesthetic.

Confirmation of a successful block

- Relief of pain.
- Anesthesia in the distribution of the blocked nerve.

Tips

- Some workers advocate drawing a line from a point 2–3 cm medial to the posterior superior iliac spine to a point 1–2 cm lateral to the sacral cornua. The sacral foraminae usually lie along this line.
- It is best to angle the X-ray beam caudally, thereby perpendicular to the sacrum, superimposing the anterior and posterior sacral foramina. Consequently, when the needle is introduced in a direction perpendicular (Fig. 4.5.8) to the skin, fluoroscopic guidance is easier. Optimally, the needle makes gentle contact with the spinal nerve in the middle of the canal (Figs 4.5.9 and 4.5.10) and produces paresthesia in the distribution of the nerve.
- While all sacral nerve roots are accessible, using this technique blockade of S5 is achieved by walking the needle caudally off the inferior edge of the bony plate of the sacrum and advancing the needle 1 cm.

Potential problems

- Caudal epidural blockade may occur with this block, but this is not a problem once low volumes are used. However, even small volumes of epidural spread may confound the diagnostic value of the block.

4.6
OCCIPITAL NERVE BLOCK

Anatomy

The greater occipital nerve arises from the dorsal rami of the second cervical nerve. From here it passes through the muscles of the neck and becomes subcutaneous at the superior nuchal line, where it emerges with the occipital artery (Fig. 4.6.1). The superior nuchal line extends from the mastoid process to the greater occipital protuberance bilaterally (Fig. 4.6.2).

Equipment

- 10 ml syringe
- 25 G needle

Fig. 4.6.1

Fig. 4.6.2

Fig. 4.6.3

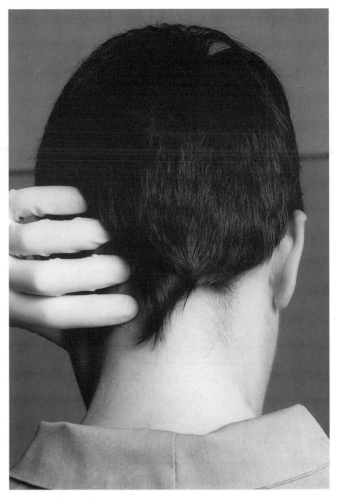

Fig. 4.6.4

- ECG, BP, and SpO$_2$ monitors
- Resuscitation equipment (see Appendix 4)

Drugs

- Lidocaine (lignocaine) 1% 10 ml (or its equivalent)
- Corticosteroid if indicated, e.g. triamcinolone 50 mg (or its equivalent)
- Resuscitation drugs (see Appendix 4)

Position of patient

- Sitting.
- Neck flexed.

Needle puncture and technique

- The superior nuchal line is cleaned with antiseptic solution (no drape is required) (Fig. 4.6.3).
- The occipital artery is palpated 2 cm lateral to the greater occipital protuberance on the superior nuchal line (Fig. 4.6.4).
- A 25 G needle is inserted subcutaneously at this point.
- After negative aspiration, 3–5 ml of lidocaine (lignocaine) 1% or its equivalent, plus corticosteroid if indicated, is injected to surround the occipital artery.
- It is often difficult to feel an occipital artery pulse. If this is the case, it is best to pick a point midway

Fig. 4.6.5

between the occipital protuberance and the mastoid bone and fan out the injection in both directions, medially and laterally from that site (Fig. 4.6.5).

Confirmation of a successful block

- Relief of pain and anesthesia in distribution of nerve.

Tips

- Bone should be contacted at a depth no greater than 1–2 cm.
- The lesser occipital nerve is blocked by redirecting the needle towards the mastoid process along the greater nuchal line and injecting a further 3 ml of solution.

Potential problems

- Injection into the cerebrospinal fluid (CSF) of the cisterna magna is possible and will produce a total spinal block.

4.7
TRIGEMINAL GANGLION (GASSERIAN) BLOCK

Anatomy

The trigeminal ganglion gives rise to the fifth cranial nerve and divides into three branches, the ophthalmic, maxillary, and mandibular nerves (Fig. 4.7.1). These provide the sensory nerve supply to the ipsilateral face and the anterior two-thirds of the head (Fig. 4.7.2). The mandibular nerve also provides motor supply to the muscles of mastication.

The trigeminal ganglion is located at the apex of the petrous temporal bone in a fold of dura mater 'Meckel's cave'. This dural invagination covers the posterior two-thirds of the ganglion and contains cerebrospinal fluid (CSF). Posterior to Meckel's cave lies the brainstem, superior to it lies the temporal lobe, and medially lies the cavernous sinus which contains the internal carotid artery and cranial nerves III, IV, and VI. Accordingly, extreme care must be taken when carrying out this block, especially if neurolytic agents are used. Blockade of the ganglion is carried out by passage of a needle through the foramen ovale, which lies immediately below it (Fig. 4.7.3).

Fig. 4.7.1

Fig. 4.7.3

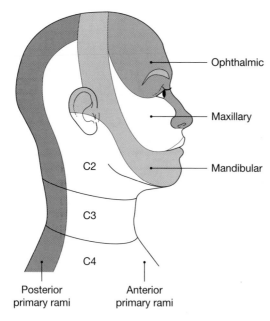

Fig. 4.7.2

Equipment

- 2 ml and 10 ml syringes
- 25 G needle
- 22 G 8–10 cm needle
- Non-ionic radio-opaque contrast medium
- ECG, BP, and SpO$_2$ monitors
- Resuscitation equipment (see Appendix 4)
- Fluoroscopy

Drugs

- Lidocaine (lignocaine) 2% 10 ml
- Lidocaine (lignocaine) 1% 10 ml (or its equivalent)
- Neurolytic agent, e.g. phenol 6% plus glycerol (or its equivalent)
- Sedative, e.g. midazolam, propofol
- Resuscitation drugs (see Appendix 4)

Position of patient

- Supine.
- Eyes directed straight ahead.

Needle puncture and technique

Caution: Injection of 0.25 ml of lidocaine (lignocaine) 1% into the CSF may result in immediate convulsion and/or loss of consciousness with possible cardiovascular system (CVS) collapse.

- The cheek on the side of the block is cleaned with antiseptic solution or saline.
- Mild sedation is induced.
- It is best to stand on the side of the block, just below the shoulder.
- The insertion point lies 1–3 cm posterior to the lateral margin of the mouth, at the medial edge of the masseter muscle (located by asking the patient to clench the jaw) and is marked.
- In edentulous patients the insertion point should be more caudad as sufficient angle towards the

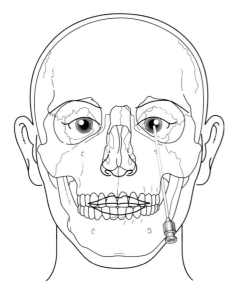

Fig. 4.7.4

infratemporal surface of the sphenoid bone may not be achieved.

■ One finger is placed inside the upper lip to avoid injection into the buccal cavity and possible bacterial contamination, and a skin wheal is raised at this site.

■ Viewed from above, a 22 G 8–10 cm needle is advanced towards the ipsilateral pupil (Figs 4.7.4, 4.7.5, 4.7.6), (or viewed from the side the needle advances towards the mid-point of the zygomatic arch (see Anatomy above) until bone is contacted; the roof of the infratemporal fossa. This lies just anterior to the foramen ovale and lateral to the base of the pterygoid process. The location of the needle tip is confirmed with fluoroscopy.

■ A depth mark is set and the needle is withdrawn to the subcutaneous tissue. With the aid of fluoroscopy the needle is reinserted to walk off the bone and enter the foramen ovale (Fig. 4.7.7).

■ Paresthesia in the distribution of the mandibular nerve (sometimes the other branches of the trigeminal nerve) or contraction of the muscles of mastication may be experienced at this point.

■ The needle is advanced a further 1 cm to bring the tip to lie in the trigeminal ganglion. The correct placement is indicated by a visible outline of Meckel's cave on injection of 0.25 ml non-ionic radio-opaque contrast medium under fluoroscopy (Figs 4.7.8 and 4.7.9).

■ The patient is allowed to awaken from sedation and is questioned about the presence and distribution of paresthesia and pain.

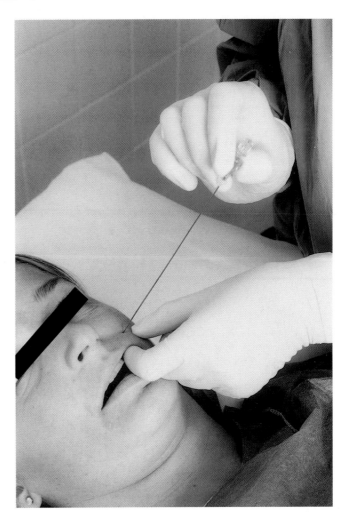

Fig. 4.7.5

■ A stimulating device may aid placement in patients who are not able to locate the paresthesia with accuracy.

■ If necessary, analgesia may be administered, although this may affect accurate assessment of the blockade.

■ Adjustment of the needle may be required to place the needle near the appropriate nerve division.

■ After careful negative aspiration for CSF or blood, lidocaine (lignocaine) 1% 0.25 ml is injected (*Caution:* injection into CSF may cause loss of consciousness). This is followed by further boluses of lidocaine (lignocaine) 1% 0.25 ml until a total of 1 ml is given.

■ After 5 minutes the patient is questioned about pain relief and changes in sensation.

■ When the desired analgesia has been achieved for diagnostic blockade the needle may be removed.

Fig. 4.7.6

Fig. 4.7.8

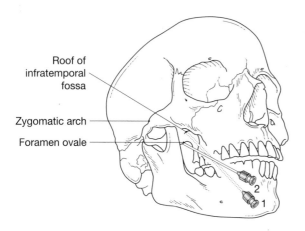

Roof of
infratemporal
fossa

Zygomatic arch

Foramen ovale

Fig. 4.7.7

Fig. 4.7.9

- When contact with the transverse process of C7 is reached, the injecting hand is steadied and the needle is withdrawn 2 mm.
- The hub of the needle is held in place with the other hand.
- After negative aspiration, lidocaine (lignocaine) 1%, 0.5 ml, is injected.
- The patient is questioned about sensation, and any change in level of consciousness is noted.
- If negative, the same procedure is repeated as 0.5 ml boluses are given until 5–8 ml is injected.
- The needle is withdrawn and the patient is immediately put in the sitting position.
- Monitors should be left attached and i.v. access left in situ for at least 30 min. Blockade of the recurrent laryngeal nerve is less likely with the C7 approach but it is wise to advise the patient not to eat or drink for 2 hours.
- Note: if aspiration of blood occurs during the block, the needle is removed and cleared, keeping the left fore- and middle fingers in place. It is then reinserted and the block is continued as above.
- If there is pain on injection and/or paresthesia, it is likely that the brachial plexus may have been contacted, the needle is withdrawn and the landmarks are rechecked.

Confirmation of successful block

- Temperature increase >1° on the side of block. The temperature should begin to rise in the finger of the blocked side within 3 minutes of injection.
- Ptosis of eyelid.
- Miosis of pupil.
- Unilateral blockage of nose on side of block.
- Unilateral flushing of conjunctiva of eye on side of block.
- Relief of sympathetically maintained pain.

Tips

- Some workers advocate targeting the ventrolateral aspect of the C7 vertebral body instead of its transverse process. The needle is directed 15–20 medially. With the aid of fluoroscopy or CT, the vertebral body is contacted just medial to the insertion of the longus colli muscle. The needle is then withdrawn 2 mm, stabilized, and 1 ml of non-ionic contrast medium is injected.
- The external jugular vein usually crosses the SCM muscle at the level of C6.
- Skin infiltration prior to block should be avoided if possible, as this will make landmarks more difficult to locate.
- An extension set may be inserted between the needle and syringe for better stability of needle (Fig. 5.2.8), but an assistant is then required to continue the procedure as described above.

Fig. 5.2.7

Fig. 5.2.8

- Lidocaine (lignocaine) 1% 10 ml may be given if a previous block failed to relieve sympathetically maintained pain in the presence of correctly placed solution. This may improve tracking of the solution caudally to produce more effective blockade of the stellate ganglion.

Potential problems

- Intra-arterial injection or intrathecal injection may result in immediate convulsion and/or loss of consciousness with possible CVS collapse.

- Hematoma may occur (avoid performing block on patients who have coagulopathy).

- Pneumothorax may occur (more likely with C7 approach).

- Recurrent laryngeal nerve block may occur and it is prudent to advise the patient about possible hoarseness post-blockade. Bilateral stellate ganglion blockade should be avoided for the same reason.

- Phrenic nerve block may occur and it is prudent to caution the patient about possible shortness of breath post blockade of the stellate ganglion.

5.3
LUMBAR SYMPATHETIC BLOCK

Anatomy

The lumbar sympathetic chain is located in the prevertebral fascia, which lies on the anterolateral aspects of the vertebral bodies. The psoas muscle separates the lumbar sympathetic chain from the lumbar somatic nerves. A single injection of local anaesthetic at the level of L2 will usually provide a complete block of postganglionic sympathetic efferents to the lower extremity because the lowest preganglionic sympathetic outflow to the chain is at the level of L2.

Equipment

- 2 ml, 5 ml and 10 ml syringes
- 30 G needle
- 15 cm 22 G needles
- Extension set (optional)
- ECG, BP, SpO_2 monitors
- Skin temperature monitor (two probes)
- Resuscitation equipment (see Appendix 4)
- Fluoroscopy

Fig. 5.3.1

Drugs

- Lidocaine (lignocaine) 1%, 5 ml for skin infiltration
- Lidocaine (lignocaine) 1%, 15–20 ml (or its equivalent) for block
- Phenol 6%
- Radio-opaque contrast medium
- Resuscitation drugs (see Appendix 4)

Position of patient

- Prone.
- Pillow under anterior superior iliac spine to flatten the normal lumbar lordosis (Fig. 5.3.1).

Needle puncture and technique

- Intravenous access is inserted.
- Monitors are attached
- Each temperature probe is attached to the plantar aspect of the big toe (Fig. 5.3.2).
- Resuscitation equipment and drugs are checked and made ready for use.
- The thoracolumbar midline and area 10 cm × 5 cm laterally is cleaned with antiseptic solution and a fenestrated drape is placed over the sterile area.
- The twelfth rib is identified and a line is drawn along its inferior border (Fig. 5.3.3).
- The iliac crests are palpated and the intercrestal line is identified (this corresponds with the inferior aspect of the spinous process of L4 or may lie in the L4–5 interspace).
- The spinous processes are counted until L2 is identified and confirmed with fluoroscopy.
- The insertion point lies 8 cm lateral to the L2 spinous process and is also marked (Fig. 5.3.4).
- A skin wheal is raised at one of the marked sites and the area is infiltrated with lidocaine (lignocaine) 1%.
- At a 30° angle to the frontal plane, a 22 G 15 cm needle is advanced in a slightly cephalad towards the lower portion of the L2 vertebral body (Fig. 5.3.5), until its vertebral body is contacted at a depth of about 7–9 cm and confirmed with fluoroscopy. If the needle contacts bone at a more superficial level, it is probable that it has come into contact with the transverse process and it will need to be repositioned.
- The needle depth is noted.

Temperature probe

Fig. 5.3.2

Fig. 5.3.3

Fig. 5.3.4

Fig. 5.3.6

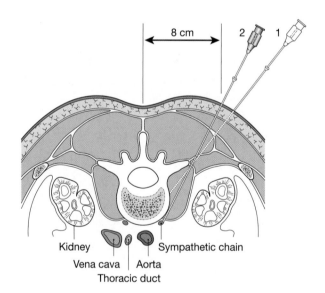

Kidney   Sympathetic chain
Vena cava   Aorta
Thoracic duct

Fig. 5.3.5

- The needle is then withdrawn to the subcutaneous tissue and, with the aid of fluoroscopy, it is re-advanced, this time at an angle 45° to the frontal plane, until the previous depth (as noted) is reached. It should slip past the vertebral body at a depth about 1–2 cm deeper than the first depth mark (Figs 5.3.5, 5.3.6).

- After negative aspiration, the fluoroscopic image is observed as a small amount of non-ionic radio-contrast medium is injected. The correct placement of the needle is indicated by the presence of a layer of contrast in a thin line along the anterior border of the vertebral column (Figs 5.3.7, 5.3.8, 5.3.9).

- After further negative aspirations, 5 ml of lidocaine (lignocaine) 1% is injected. The patient is questioned about pain relief and observations of skin temperature are made. There should be little resistance to injection, similar to resistance felt when injecting through an epidural needle. If resistance is encountered, or if the injection is painful, the needle should be repositioned. A unilateral rise in skin temperature indicates a successful block.

- After 10 minutes the patient is questioned about pain relief and any symptoms of somatic nerve blockade. Sensory and motor functioning of the lower extremities is checked. The procedure should be abandoned if there is evidence of somatic blockade.

- Neurolysis may be achieved by leaving the needle in place after block has been confirmed and injecting 5 ml phenol 6%. To avoid leaving alcohol in the needle tract, the needle is then cleared with air or local anesthetic 1 ml, and removed. However, because

Fig. 5.4.7

Fig. 5.4.9

Fig. 5.4.8

- The thoracolumbar midline and area 10 cm × 5 cm laterally is cleaned with antiseptic solution and a fenestrated drape is placed over the sterile area.

- The twelfth rib is identified and a line is drawn along its inferior border.

- The iliac crests are palpated and the intercrestal line is identified (this corresponds with the inferior aspect of the spinous process of L4 or may lie in the L4–5 interspace).

- The spinous processes are counted until L1 is identified and confirmed with fluoroscopy.

- The insertion points lie about 8 cm lateral to the L2 spinous process at the lower border of the twelfth rib and are also marked (Fig. 5.4.5).

- A skin wheal is raised at one of the marked sites and the area is infiltrated with lidocaine (lignocaine) 1%.

- At a 45° angle to the frontal plane a 22 G 15 cm needle is advanced in a slightly cephalad direction (Figs 5.4.6, 5.4.7, 5.4.8) until the vertebral body of L1 is contacted at a depth of about 7–9 cm (Figs 5.4.9,

Fig. 5.4.10

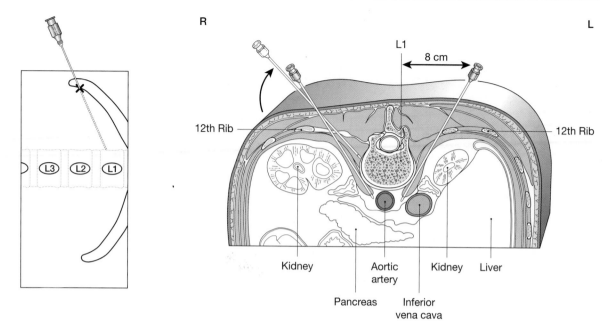

R   L

L1

8 cm

12th Rib   12th Rib

Kidney   Aortic   Kidney   Liver
artery

Pancreas   Inferior
vena cava

Fig. 5.4.11

a   b

Fig. 5.4.12a,b

and 5.4.10) and confirmed with fluoroscopy. If the needle contacts bone at a more superficial level, it is probable that it has come into contact with the transverse process and needs to be repositioned.

- The needle depth is noted.
- The needle is then withdrawn to the subcutaneous tissue and, with the aid of fluoroscopy, it is re-advanced at a greater angle so as to glide past the vertebral body. It should slip past the vertebral body at a depth about 1–2 cm deeper than the first depth mark. (Fig. 5.4.11)
- After negative aspiration, the fluoroscopic image is observed as a small amount of non-ionic radio-contrast medium is injected. The correct placement of the needle is indicated by the presence of a layer of contrast in a thin line along the anterior border of the vertebral column. This should have a similar radiologic appearance as placement of non-ionic radio-contrast medium anterior to the body of L2 in lumbar sympathetic blockade (Figs 5.4.12 a,b).
- The procedure is repeated on the other side, in a mirrored fashion. (Fig. 5.4.13)
- On the left side advancement usually results in perforation of the aorta. If this occurs advancing the needle through the aorta usually places the needle within the plexus.
- After further negative aspirations, 5 ml of lidocaine (lignocaine) 1% is injected bilaterally. There should be

little resistance to injection, similar to resistance felt when injecting through an epidural needle. If resistance is encountered, or if the injection is painful, the needles should be repositioned.

- After 10 minutes the patient is questioned about pain relief and any symptoms of somatic nerve blockade. Sensory and motor functioning of the lower extremities is checked. The procedure should be abandoned if there is evidence of somatic blockade.
- After further aspiration, 5 ml boluses of lidocaine (lignocaine) 1% (or its equivalent) are injected until a total of 10 ml is reached on each side.
- After confirmation of pain relief and lack of somatic block, 20 ml of alcohol 50% is injected through each needle using glass syringes. Injection through a plastic syringe can be difficult as alcohol may dissolve the rubber plunger. Phenol 10% may also be used with similar efficacy. To avoid leaving alcohol in the needle tract the needles are then cleared with air or local anesthetic 1 ml, and removed.
- Monitors should be left attached and i.v. access left in situ for at least 30 min.

Confirmation of a successful block

- Relief of upper abdominal pain.

Tips

- After injection of non-ionic radio-contrast medium, a blush will indicate injection into muscle. If visible contrast medium disappears immediately it is likely that intravascular injection has occurred.
- Consideration should be given to performance of the block under CT control if the block is unsuccessful.
- Placement of the needle anterior to the diaphragmatic crus can also be achieved via insertion through the abdominal wall.

Potential problems

- The position of each needle tip should always be confirmed with fluoroscopy before injection of neurolytic agent as it may lie in the peritoneal cavity, within a viscus or intravascularly. If a needle tip is placed too superficially, the tip may come to lie in the intervertebral foramen and injection may result in an epidural block or a somatic nerve block. Injection of neurolytic solution into the psoas muscle may cause rhabdomyolysis.

Fig. 5.4.13

- Perforation of the aorta or the inferior vena cava is possible and consequently the block should be avoided in patients with coagulopathy. Dissection of the aorta may occur as a result of direct damage during the block. Retroperitoneal hematoma may occur and for this reason also the block should be avoided in patients with coagulopathy.
- Orthostatic hypotension may occur as a result of sympathetic blockade for up to 3 days after a neurolytic block. Diarrhea may occur also and hydration of the patient should be monitored.
- Pneumothorax may occur.
- Transient motor paralysis and paraplegia may occur after the block, probably as a result of spasm of the segmental arteries.

- Perforation of the intervertebral disc may occur, but this also is usually of no clinical significance.
- Perforation of the kidney or ureter is usually of no clinical significance unless neurolytic agent is injected.
- The thoracic duct may be damaged (possibly causing chylothorax, or lymphedema).
- Abdominal and chest discomfort may be experienced for 30 minutes after injection of alcohol.
- There may be a detectable odor from the breath after alcohol injection.
- Patients in the prone positioned should be monitored carefully when intravenous sedation is administered.

5.5
CELIAC PLEXUS BLOCK—ANTEROCRURAL APPROACH

Anatomy

The anterocrural approach places a needle anterior to the crus of the right side of the diaphragm. The needle is inserted more medially and directed at a larger angle towards the midline until it comes to lie in the retroperitoneal compartment between the aorta, and the inferior vena cava dorsally, and the pancreas ventrally (Fig. 5.5.1). Fluoroscopic imaging is necessary for accurate placement of the single anterocrural needle using this approach.

Equipment

- 2 ml, 5 ml and 10 ml syringes
- 30 G needle
- 15 cm 20 G needle (penetration of the diaphragmatic crus is easier with a large gauge needle)
- Extension set (optional)
- ECG, BP, SpO$_2$ monitors
- Resuscitation equipment (see Appendix 4)
- Fluoroscopy

Drugs

- Mild sedative
- Lidocaine (lignocaine) 1%, 5 ml for skin infiltration

- Lidocaine (lignocaine) 1%, 15–20 ml (or its equivalent) for block
- Alcohol 50% or phenol 10%
- Non-ionic radio-opaque contrast medium
- Resuscitation drugs (see Appendix 4)

Position of patient

- Prone.
- Pillow under anterior superior iliac spine to flatten the normal lumbar lordosis (Fig. 5.5.2).

Needle puncture and technique

- Intravenous access is inserted.
- Monitors are attached.
- Resuscitation equipment and drugs are checked and made ready for use.
- Mild sedation may be induced.
- The thoracolumbar midline and area 10 cm × 5 cm laterally is cleaned with antiseptic solution and a fenestrated drape is placed over the sterile area.
- The twelfth rib is identified and a line is drawn along its inferior border.

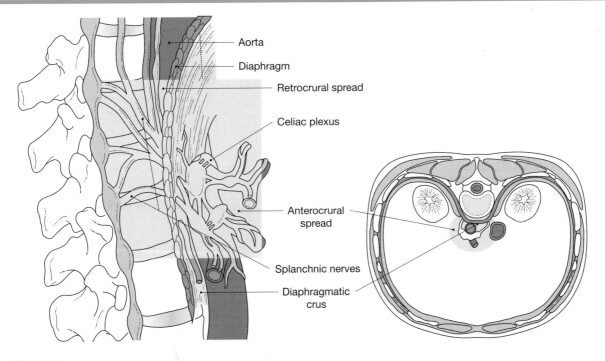

Aorta

Diaphragm

Retrocrural spread

Celiac plexus

Anterocrural
spread

Splanchnic nerves

Diaphragmatic
crus

Fig. 5.5.1a

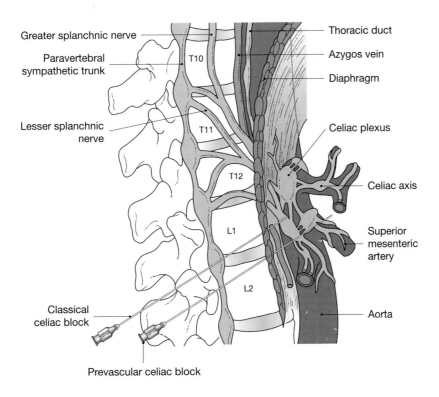

Greater splanchnic nerve

Paravertebral
sympathetic trunk

Lesser splanchnic
nerve

T10

T11

T12

L1

L2

Thoracic duct

Azygos vein

Diaphragm

Celiac plexus

Celiac axis

Superior
mesenteric
artery

Aorta

Classical
celiac block

Prevascular celiac block

Fig. 5.5.1b

Fig. 5.5.2

- The iliac crests are palpated and the intercrestal line is identified (this corresponds with the inferior aspect of the spinous process of L4 or may lie in the L4–5 interspace).
- The spinous processes are counted until L1 is identified and confirmed with fluoroscopy.
- The insertion point lies about 5 cm lateral to the L1 spinous process at the lower border of the twelfth rib on the right and is also marked.
- A skin wheal is raised at one of the marked sites and the area is infiltrated with lidocaine (lignocaine) 1%.

- At a 60° angle to the frontal plane a 20 G 15 cm needle is advanced in a slightly cephalad direction until the vertebral body is contacted at a depth of about 7–9 cm (Fig. 5.5.3) and confirmed with fluoroscopy. If the needle contacts bone at a more superficial level, it is probable that it has come into contact with the transverse process and needs to be repositioned.
- The needle depth is noted.
- The needle is then withdrawn to the subcutaneous tissue, and with the aid of fluoroscopy it is re-advanced at a greater angle so as to glide past the

Fig. 5.5.3

Fig. 5.5.4

vertebral body. It should slip past the vertebral body at a depth about 1–2 cm deeper than the first depth mark.

- After negative aspiration, the fluoroscopic image is observed as a small amount of non-ionic radio-contrast medium is injected. The correct placement of the needle is indicated by the presence of a layer of contrast in a thin line along the anterior border of the vertebral column. This should have a similar radiologic appearance as placement of non-ionic radio-contrast medium anterior to the vetebral body of L2 as in lumbar sympathetic blockade (Fig. 5.5.4).

- After further negative aspirations, 5 ml of lidocaine (lignocaine) 1% is injected. There should be little resistance to injection, similar to that felt when injecting through an epidural needle. If resistance is encountered, or if the injection is painful, the needles should be repositioned.

- After 10 minutes the patient is questioned about pain relief and any symptoms of somatic nerve blockade. Sensory and motor functioning of the lower extremities is checked. The procedure should be abandoned if there is evidence of somatic blockade.

- After further aspiration, boluses of 5 ml of lidocaine (lignocaine) 1%, (or its equivalent) are injected until a total of 10 ml is reached on each side.

- After confirmation of pain relief and lack of somatic block, 30 ml of alcohol 50% is injected through the needle using glass syringes. Injection through a plastic syringe can be difficult as alcohol may dissolve the rubber plunger. Phenol 10% may also be used with similar efficacy.

- To avoid leaving alcohol in the needle tract the needle is then cleared with air or local anesthetic 1 ml, and removed.

- Monitors should be left attached and i.v. access left in situ for at least 30 min.

Fig. 5.5.5

Confirmation of a successful block

Relief of upper abdominal pain.

Tips

- After injection of non-ionic radio-contrast medium, a blush will indicate injection into muscle. If visible contrast medium disappears immediately it is likely that intravascular injection has occurred.
- Consideration should be given to performance of the block under CT control if the block is unsuccessful.
- Placement of the needle anterior to the diaphragmatic crus can also be achieved via insertion through the abdominal wall (Fig. 5.5.5).

Potential problems

- The position of each needle tip should always be confirmed with fluoroscopy prior to injection of neurolytic agent as it may lie in the peritoneal cavity, within a viscus or intravascularly. If a needle tip is placed too superficially, the tip may come to lie in the intervertebral foramen and injection may result in epidural block or a somatic nerve block. Injection of neurolytic solution into the psoas muscle may cause rhabdomyolysis.
- Perforation of the aorta or the inferior vena cava is possible and consequently the block should be avoided in patients with coagulopathy. Dissection of the aorta may occur as a result of direct damage during the block. Retroperitoneal hematoma may occur and for this reason also the block should be avoided in patients with coagulopathy.
- Orthostatic hypotension may occur as a result of sympathetic blockade for up to three days after a neurolytic block. Diarrhea may occur also and hydration of the patient should be monitored.
- Pneumothorax may occur.
- Transient motor paralysis and paraplegia may occur after the block, probably as a result of spasm of segmental arteries.
- Perforation of the intervertebral disc may occur, but this also is usually of no clinical significance.
- Perforation of the kidney or ureter is usually of no clinical significance unless neurolytic agents are injected.
- The thoracic duct may be damaged (possibly causing chylothorax, or lymphedema).
- Abdominal and chest discomfort may be experienced for 30 minutes after injection of alcohol.
- There may be a detectable odor from the breath after alcohol injection.
- Patients in the prone positioned should be monitored carefully when intravenous sedation is administered.

5.6 SPLANCHNIC NERVE BLOCK

Anatomy

The greater splanchnic nerve arises from the T5/6–T9/10 nerve roots; the lesser splanchnic nerve arises from the T10/11 nerve roots; the least splanchnic nerve arises from the T11 and T12 nerve roots. These three nerves pass in the paravertebral space through the diaphragmatic crus to the celiac ganglia. All three splanchnic nerves are preganglionic. After synapsing in the paired celiac ganglia, postganglionic fibers innervate the abdominal visceral organs via the celiac plexus (Fig. 5.6.1) (see Fig. 5.4.2b).

The compartment in which the splanchnic nerves lie is very narrow laterally, necessitating placement of needle tips very close to the vertebral bodies of the T11 or T12 vertebrae. The technique of placement is similar to that for celiac plexus blockade.

Equipment

- 2 ml, 5 ml and 10 ml syringes
- 30 G needle
- Two 15 cm 20 G needles
- Extension set (optional)
- ECG, BP, SpO_2 monitors
- Resuscitation equipment (see Appendix 4)
- Fluoroscopy

Drugs

- Lidocaine (lignocaine) 1%, 5 ml for skin infiltration

Fig. 5.9.1

Fig. 5.9.2

Position of patient

■ Supine.

Technique

■ Intravenous access is inserted in contralateral limb.

■ Peripheral i.v. access is inserted in the limb to be blocked.

■ Monitors are attached.

■ Resuscitation equipment and drugs are checked and made ready for use.

■ The limb is raised above the level of the heart for 2 min (Fig. 5.9.1).

■ With the limb raised, it is exsanguinated by applying a tight wrap, e.g. Esmarch bandage.

■ A thin layer of padding is applied, e.g. Velband, under the tourniquet site.

■ The tourniquet is applied and the cuff is inflated to a pressure 100 mmHg higher than the systolic blood pressure (Fig. 5.9.2).

■ The limb is then lowered. A mixture of lidocaine (lignocaine) 0.5% 15 ml (*without epinephrine (adrenaline)* bretylium 1.5 mg/kg (or guanethidine 0.25 mg/kg), and NaCl to make a total volume of 40 ml (a final lidocaine (lignocaine) solution of 0.25%), is injected through the i.v. cannula in the affected limb.

Temperature probe

Fig. 5.9.3

■ The tourniquet is allowed to remain inflated for at least 30 min.

■ It is then deflated in one step, but left in place. Re-inflation may be required if there is a precipitous change in blood pressure.

■ Monitors should be left attached and i.v. access left in situ for at least 30 min.

Fig. 5.9.4

Fig. 5.9.6

Fig. 5.9.5

Fig. 5.9.7

Confirmation of a successful block

- Relief of sympathetically maintained pain.
- Measurements of skin temperature of the affected limb before and after the block should demonstrate temperature increase. However, the sympatholytic effect of the drug may not be immediate (Fig. 5.9.3).

Tips

- If i.v. access to the affected limb is difficult due to vasoconstriction, a smear of glycerol trinitrate cream on the dorsum of the hand will usually aid i.v. insertion.
- A single or double cuff may be employed for this block but a double tourniquet may make the block more comfortable. The proximal cuff is inflated first. A few minutes after injection the distal cuff is inflated and when inflation is complete the proximal cuff is released.
- Retrograde cannulation, i.e. towards the periphery (Figs 5.9.4, 5.9.5) rather than proximally (Figs 5.9.6, 5.9.7), may help direct the spread of bretylium to the periphery.
- Active or passive movements of the limb may hasten the distribution of bretylium to the periphery.

- If the tourniquet inflation is painful, inhalation of nitrous oxide–oxygen mixture may improve comfort.
- Repeated blocks may bring about gradual improvement in sympathetically maintained pain.
- Immediate physiotherapy after block may improve outcome.

Potential problems

- Accidental deflation of the tourniquet early in the procedure may cause a precipitous rise in blood pressure due to the general release of endogenous norepinephrine when unfixed bretylium enters the circulation. Systemic toxicity of lidocaine (lignocaine) may also occur, possibly causing seizures. Blood pressure may decrease after deflation of the cuff later in the procedure.
- The tourniquet inflation may be painful.
- A sensation of burning may occur after injection due to release of endogenous norepinephrine.
- Neuropraxia may occur (rarely) with a very tight tourniquet.
- Avoid in sickle cell anemia.

5.10
INTRAVENOUS REGIONAL SYMPATHETIC BLOCK—LOWER LIMB

Anatomy

As in the case of the upper limb, peripheral sympathetic blockade is achieved by limiting the effect of the sympatholytic agent to the tissues of the affected limb using a tourniquet. Intravenous injection of an agent releases endogenous norepinephrine from sympathetic nerve endings, which causes depletion of this neurotransmitter, and may bring about a chemical sympathetic block.

Equipment

- 50 ml syringe
- Two i.v. cannulae
- Pneumatic tourniquet
- ECG, BP and SpO$_2$ monitors
- Skin temperature monitor
- Resuscitation equipment (see Appendix 4)

Drugs

- Lidocaine (lignocaine) 0.5% *without adrenaline/epinephrine*, or its equivalent
- Bretylium 1.5 mg/kg (or its equivalent, e.g. guanethedine 0.5 mg/kg)
- Saline (NaCl) 30 ml
- Resuscitation drugs (see Appendix 4)

Position of patient

- Supine.

Technique

- Intravenous access is inserted in contralateral limb.
- Peripheral i.v. access is inserted in the limb to be blocked.
- Monitors are attached.
- Resuscitation equipment and drugs are checked and made ready for use.
- The limb is raised above the level of the heart for 2 min (Fig. 5.10.1).

Fig. 5.10.1

Fig. 5.10.2

- With the limb raised, it is exsanguinated by applying a tight wrap, e.g. Esmarch bandage (Fig. 5.10.2).
- A thin layer of padding is applied, e.g. Velband, under the tourniquet site.
- The tourniquet is applied and inflated to a pressure 100 mmHg higher than the systolic blood pressure. A second tourniquet may be applied to the calf of patients with no known predispositions to deep venous thrombosis. Inflation of this second cuff may

Single cuff

Fig. 5.10.3

Temperature probe

Fig. 5.10.4

aid limitation of spread of sympatholytic agent to the periphery (Fig. 5.10.3).

■ The limb is then lowered and a mixture of lidocaine (lignocaine) 0.5% 25 ml *(without* epinephrine/adrenaline)*, bretylium 1.5 mg/kg (or its equivalent) and NaCl to make a total volume of 40 ml (a final lidocaine (lignocaine) solution of 0.25%) is injected through the i.v. cannula in the affected limb.

■ The tourniquet is allowed to remain inflated for at least 30 min.

■ It is then deflated in one step, but left in place. Re-inflation may be required if there is a precipitous change in blood pressure.

■ Monitors should be left attached and i.v. access left in situ for at least 30 min.

Confirmation of a successful block

■ Relief of sympathetically maintained pain.

■ Measurements of skin temperature of the affected limb before and after the block should demonstrate temperature increase.

Tips

■ Retrograde cannulation may be carried out to aid delivery of the drug to the periphery (Fig. 5.10.5).

■ See also Tips listed in Section 5.9

Fig. 5.10.5

Potential problems

■ Accidental deflation of the tourniquet early in the procedure may cause a precipitous rise in blood pressure due to the general release of endogenous norepinephrine or epinephrine when unfixed bretylium enters the circulation. Systemic toxicity of lidocaine (lignocaine) may also occur in high doses possibly causing seizures. Blood pressure may decrease after deflation of the cuff later in the procedure.

- The tourniquet inflation may be painful.
- A sensation of burning may occur after injection due to release of endogenous norepinephrine.

- Neuropraxia may occur (rarely) with a very tight tourniquet.
- Avoid in sickle cell anemia.

Chapter 6

Muscle injections

Myofascial pain occurs commonly in the muscles of the upper and lower back. It is characterized by pain associated with movement of the affected muscles that develop areas of extreme tenderness, termed trigger points. Palpation of these points is usually perceived as a tight band or firm nodule in the muscle and reproduces pain that may be referred some distance from the site of palpation. Involuntary muscular contraction can occur on palpation, and snapping palpation can result in a local twitch response. Electromyography (EMG) is not reliable in diagnosing myofascial pain syndrome and it is worth remembering that this syndrome may occur in association with underlying painful disorders of the spine.

Injection of trigger points with local anaesthetic, especially if repeated several times and combined with stretching exercises, may have a beneficial therapeutic effect on the pain of myofascial pain syndrome. Pain reproduction during injection, followed by relief of pain after injection, that lasts at least as long as the expected local anaesthetic effect, indicates that these painful points contribute to myofascial pain syndrome.

Fibromyalgia is a pain syndrome characterized by widespread, diffuse and usually symmetrical tender areas of muscles. Bony structures, such as costochondral junctions and lateral epicondyles, produce local pain, but not referred, on palpation of tender points. Injection of these tender areas typically does not improve the pain of fibromyalgia.

Usually a dilute solution of local anaesthetic suffices for beneficial effect. Bupivacaine produces more muscle degeneration than any other local anaesthetic when injected into a muscle, and consequently it is usually avoided, lidocaine (lignocaine) being the usual local anaesthetic of choice.

The optimum number of trigger-point injections required to produce pain relief is variable. The injection sites may themselves be painful after the local anaesthetic wears off. This may exacerbate muscle spasm if too many trigger-point injections are performed. Consideration should be given to the severity of the muscle spasm, the number of trigger points and to the sensitivity of the patient to pain when deciding on the number of injections.

6.1
TRIGGER-POINT INJECTIONS—NECK AND THORAX

Anatomy

The muscles most often involved in myofascial pain syndrome of the neck include the trapezius, rhomboid minor and major, latissimus dorsi, levator scapulae and splenius capitis (Fig. 6.1.1; see also Fig. 2.1.2).

Equipment

- 10 ml syringe
- 25 G needle

Drugs

- Lidocaine (lignocaine) 0.5% 10 ml

Position of patient

- Prone
- Pillow under chest to allow the neck to flex.
- The sitting position is also used, but vasovagal response may follow trigger-point injections especially in young adults, and it is probably more prudent to use the prone position.

Needle puncture and technique

- The neck, shoulders and upper posterior thorax are cleaned with antiseptic solution.
- Trigger points in the muscles are palpated (Fig. 6.1.2) and marked (Fig. 6.1.3).

Fig. 6.1.1

Fig. 6.1.2

Fig. 6.1.3

Fig. 6.1.4

- A 25 G needle with syringe attached is inserted into a trigger point (Fig. 6.1.4).

- After negative aspiration, 2–3 ml of lidocaine (lignocaine) 0.5% is injected into the trigger point while moving the needle back and forth through the muscle.

- After injection, the next trigger point is injected in the same manner (Fig. 6.1.5 a,b).

Confirmation of a successful injection

- Pain reproduction when the needle enters the muscle confirms correct placement.

Fig. 6.1.5a

Fig. 6.1.6

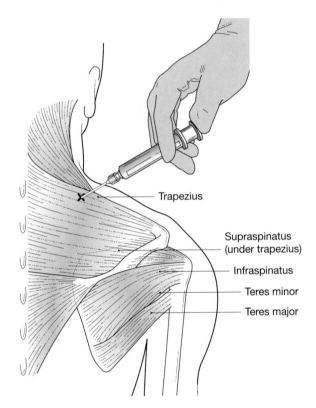

Trapezius

Supraspinatus
(under trapezius)

Infraspinatus

Teres minor

Teres major

Fig. 6.1.5b

Tips

- For best results, injection is carried out in a fan-like manner by repeatedly withdrawing the needle slightly and redirecting it (Fig. 6.1.6).
- Stretching of the involved muscles by physiotherapy within the duration of the local anesthesia improves results.
- Some workers advocate massage of the area immediately after injection.

Potential problems

- Pain on injection.
- Vasovagal response (especially in young adults in the sitting position).
- Pneumothorax (especially in thin patients).

6.2
TRIGGER-POINT INJECTIONS—BACK

Anatomy

The muscles most often involved in myofascial pain syndrome of the back include the erector spinae (the longissimus, iliocostalis and spinalis columns) and the deep transversospinal (semispinalis, multifidus and rotarores) muscles (Fig. 6.2.1a,b). In the buttocks, spasm of the gluteus medius muscle may also cause significant pain.

Equipment

- 10 ml syringe
- 25 G needle

Drugs

- Lidocaine (lignocaine) 0.5% 10 ml

Position of patient

- Prone.
- Pillow under abdomen to straighten the normal lumbar lordosis (Fig. 6.2.2 a).

- The sitting position is also used, but vasovagal response may follow trigger-point injections, and it is probably more prudent to use the prone position.
- Alternatively, the semiprone position will also allow access to affected muscles (Fig. 6.2.2 b).

Needle puncture and technique

- The midline and the surrounding area are cleaned with antiseptic solution.
- Trigger points in the muscles are identified by palpation and marked (Fig. 6.2.3).
- A 25 G needle with syringe attached is inserted into a trigger point (Fig. 6.2.4).
- After negative aspiration, 2–3 ml of lidocaine (lignocaine) 0.5% is injected into the trigger point while moving the needle back and forth through the muscle (Fig. 6.2.5).
- After injection, the next trigger point is injected in the same manner.

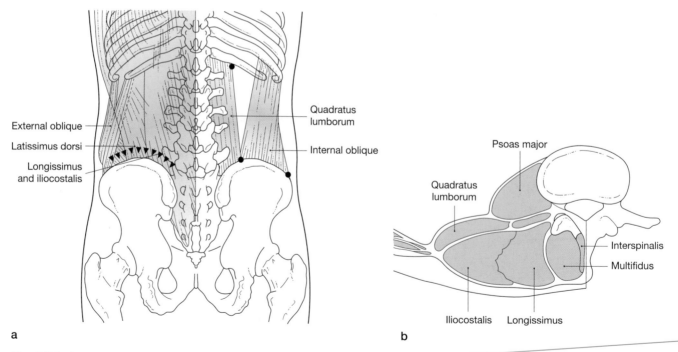

External oblique

Latissimus dorsi

Longissimus and iliocostalis

Quadratus lumborum

Internal oblique

Psoas major

Quadratus lumborum

Interspinalis

Multifidus

Iliocostalis   Longissimus

a

b

Fig. 6.2.1a,b

a

b

Fig. 6.2.2a,b

Fig. 6.2.3

Fig. 6.2.4

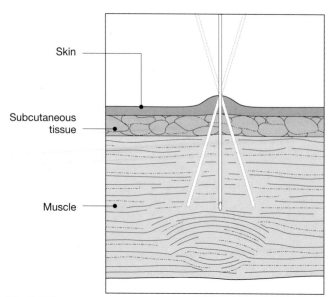

Skin

Subcutaneous
tissue

Muscle

Fig. 6.2.5

Confirmation of a successful injection

■ Pain reproduction when the needle enters the muscle confirms correct placement.

Tips

■ For best results, injection is carried out in a fan-like manner by repeatedly withdrawing the needle slightly and redirecting it.

■ Stretching of the involved muscles by physiotherapy within the duration of the local anaesthetic improves results.

■ Some workers advocate massage of the area immediately after injection.

Potential problems

■ Pain on injection.

■ Vasovagal response (especially young adults in the sitting position).

■ Pneumothorax (especially in thin patients) is also a possibility when injecting the upper back.

6.3
GLUTEUS MEDIUS INJECTION

Anatomy

When the buttock muscles are relaxed the quadratus femoris, gemelli and gluteus medius muscles can be palpated. Spasm of the gluteus medius muscle (Fig. 6.3.1) may be the source of buttock pain and may respond to trigger-point injection. Unlike pirformis muscle spasm, this does not produce symptoms of sciatic nerve irritation but causes localized pain, often referred to the posterior thigh and calf.

Equipment

- 10 ml syringe
- 22 G needle

Drugs

- Lidocaine (lignocaine) 0.5% 10 ml

Position of patient

- Prone.
- Pillow under abdomen to flatten the normal lumbar lordosis Fig. 6.3.2).

Needle puncture and technique

- The surface of the buttock and hip is cleaned with antiseptic solution.

Fig. 6.3.3

Fig. 6.3.1

Fig. 6.3.2

Fig. 6.3.4

Gluteus medius

Fig. 6.3.6

Fig. 6.3.5

- The posterior superior iliac spine is palpated and marked.
- The greater trochanter is palpated.
- The insertion point of the needle lies approximately 2 cm medial and superior to the greater trochanter (Figs 6.3.3, 6.3.4).
- A 22 G needle is introduced in a direction vertical to the skin and advanced until it is felt to be gripped by the tense muscle (Fig. 6.3.5).
- After negative aspiration, lidocaine (lignocaine) 1% 3 ml is injected in the substance of the muscle while moving the needle back and forth in the muscle (Fig. 6.3.6).

- The procedure is repeated if other trigger points are present in the muscle.

Confirmation of a successful injection

- Pain reproduction when the needle enters the muscle confirms correct placement of the needle.
- Relief of pain on abduction of the hip.

Tips

- For best results injection is carried out in a fan-like manner by repeatedly withdrawing the needle slightly and redirecting it (see inset in Fig. 6.3.6).

Potential problems

- Sciatic nerve block; although this is unusual because the injection site is not very close to the sciatic notch, it is prudent to warn patient of the possibility.
- Infection or abscess formation.

6.4
PIRIFORMIS INJECTION

Anatomy

The piriformis muscle inserts into the pelvic surface of the sacrum from the second to the fourth segments, lateral to the anterior sacral foramina, and passes out of the pelvis through the greater sciatic foramen to insert into the superior aspect of the greater trochanter (Fig. 6.4.1). It overlies the sciatic nerve in the greater sciatic foramen. Contraction contributes to abduction of the lower limb. Spasm of the muscle in myofascial pain syndrome often causes pain referred to the posterior thigh and calf.

Equipment

■ 2 ml syringe and two 5 ml syringes

■ 25 G needle

■ 22 G spinal needle, end-opening

Drugs

■ Lidocaine (lignocaine) 1% 10 ml (or its equivalent)

Position of patient

■ Prone.

■ Pillow under abdomen to flatten the normal lumbar lordosis (Fig. 6.4.2).

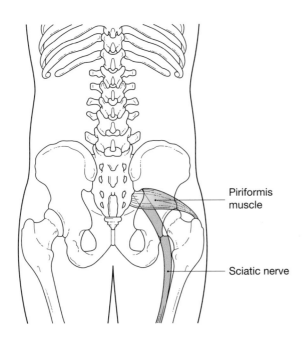

Piriformis muscle

Sciatic nerve

Fig. 6.4.1

Fig. 6.4.2

a

b

c

Fig. 6.4.3a,b,c

Fig. 6.4.4

Needle puncture and technique

- The surface of the buttock and hip is cleaned with antiseptic solution and a fenestrated drape is placed over the sterile area.

- The posterior superior iliac spine is palpated and marked.

- The greater trochanter is palpated and marked.

- The insertion points of the needle lie at the points one-third and two-thirds along, and 1–3 cm below the line connecting these two marks (Figs 6.4.3 a,b,c).

- The first insertion point, the medial one, is infiltrated with lidocaine (lignocaine) 1% 2 ml.

- A 22 G spinal needle is introduced in a direction vertical to the skin and advanced until it is felt to be

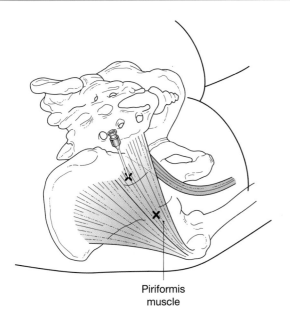

Piriformis
muscle

Fig. 6.4.5

gripped by the tense piriformis muscle, or until bone is contacted (Figs 6.4.4, 6.4.5).

■ The end-point is a fascial click at a depth of about 4–5 cm, depending on the thickness of adipose tissue.

■ The patient is questioned about the presence of pain, paresthesia, and changes in sensation in the distribution of the sciatic nerve, while the needle is being advanced.

■ If these symptoms arise, the needle may be in contact with the sciatic nerve and should be repositioned. It is also possible that spasm of the muscle on needle insertion may produce these symptoms and often reproduction of pain occurs with entry into the muscle.

■ After negative aspiration, lidocaine (lignocaine) 1% 5 ml is injected.

Confirmation of a successful injection

■ Relief of pain on abduction of the lower limb against pressure on the lateral knee in the sitting position.

Tips

■ If injection is not successful in relieving the pain, it may be repeated at the lateral insertion point. This lies at a point two-thirds along and 1–3 cm below the line joining the posterior superior iliac spine and the greater trochanter.

Potential problems

■ Sciatic nerve block.
■ Infection or abscess may occur (rarely).

Chapter 7

Transcutaneous electrical nerve stimulation (TENS)

Transcutaneous electrical nerve stimulation is thought to modify pain appreciation by stimulation of large fibers thereby blocking (or 'closing the gate' to) smaller C fibers carrying nociceptive impulses. There is also evidence that high-frequency stimulation of the skin increases latency and decreases maximum firing rates in small afferent fibers. This can produce conduction blockade in C fibers as the current is increased, probably via potassium efflux from the axon. It is thought that a combination of these actions is responsible for the analgesia derived from the use of TENS. This is probably not related to opiate-mediated mechanisms when conventional parameters are used.

Not all pain responds to TENS. If the usual parameters do not produce pain relief, low frequency, high intensity stimulation may be tried. This means that the current amplitude is increased to a level that produces mild discomfort and muscle stimulation. Analgesia from this type of stimulation may be due to opiate-mediated mechanisms. Burst stimulation means short bursts of high frequency stimulation delivered at 1–2 Hz and may also relieve pain that is not responsive to conventional TENS.

A TENS trial may be carried out prior to giving the unit to the patient to use at home. This allows the patient to become familiar with the use of TENS, and to ensure that the pain is not aggravated by its use. A minimum of one hour is recommended as the trial period. This will indicate whether the patient is likely to respond to TENS. However, failure to respond within this time period does not necessarily mean that there will be no response if used for longer periods, or with different settings. It is important to allow the patient to use the TENS at home for a period of at least 14 days.

The TENS stimulator is a battery-operated pulse generator which has several controls (Fig. 7.1.1 a,b). These include an on/off switch plus amplitude control, frequency control, mode selector and width control. In addition, multichannel units have amplitude controls for each channel. The pulse generator connects to leads that then connect to electrodes, which are applied to the skin. Electrodes are applied in pairs (Figs 7.1.2, 7.1.3), and are positioned so that they lie along the direction of the nerves in the area being treated, e.g. longitudinally in the limbs, but dermatomally in the trunk.

a

b

Fig. 7.1.1a,b

Fig. 7.1.2

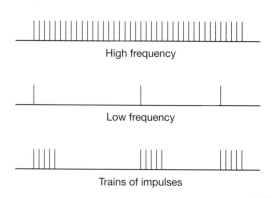

Fig. 7.1.3

Control settings (Figs 7.1.4, 7.1.5)

Continuous stimulation

- Amplitude set to zero.
- Pulse width set to midrange.

- Switch to continuous mode.
- Increase pulse amplitude level gradually to the maximum level for comfort (sensation should be strong but not painful).
- Adjust pulse frequency to maximum level for comfort (amplitude may be reduced as pulse width is increased).
- Adjust pulse width to maximum level for comfort.
- Maintain for 45–60 min.

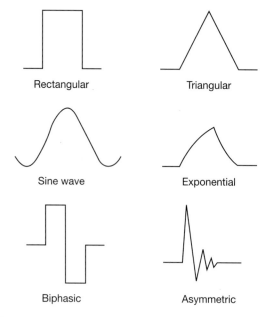

Rectangular

Triangular

Sine wave

Exponential

Biphasic

Asymmetric

Fig. 7.1.4

High frequency

Low frequency

Trains of impulses

Fig. 7.1.5

Modulated settings

Burst stimulation

- All controls set to zero.
- Switch to pulsed mode.
- Frequency set to 1–2 Hz.
- Increase amplitude and pulse width as with continuous mode described above.
- Maintain for 45–60 min.

Low-frequency high-intensity stimulation

- All controls set to zero.
- Increase amplitude to level where the muscle underlying the electrodes twitches visibly but not painfully.
- Increase frequency to 2–4 Hz.
- Maintain for short period (5–15 min).

All the types of stimulation should be tried for each pain, and the effects on the pain should be compared. The optimum parameters must be found by trial and error. The patient is usually advised to begin by using TENS for at least one hour three times a day. Once the effect of TENS on the pain is known it is recommended that stimulation should be discontinued after 30 minutes if the patient experiences one or more hours of analgesia from a single application. If pain relief is achieved only during stimulation, the unit can be kept on constantly. However, electrode sites should be changed every 24 hours. Occasionally, skin rash under the electrodes may occur and this problem may be minimized by frequent rotation of the electrode sites and with topical steroids. However, very few side effects are associated with the use of TENS. Electrical skin burns may occur if TENS is applied to skin with poor innervation and it is necessary to ensure that there is normal sensation prior to applying the electrodes. Allergic reaction to the electrodes or the adhesive tape has also been described, but is not common.

Use of TENS is contraindicated on areas over the anterior neck (stimulation of carotid sinus, larynx), over the pregnant uterus or in the presence of a cardiac pacemaker.

Note: Description of the insertion technique of a spinal cord stimulator is outside the scope of this text as the techniques are specific to the different types of stimulator.

Appendix 1   Suggested local anesthetics

Drug name	Duration of action	Onset of action	Recommended maximum dose
Lidocaine (lignocaine)	1–2 h	fast	3 mg/kg
Levobupivacaine	2–4 h	slow	4 mg/kg
Bupivacaine	2–4 h	slow	2 mg/kg
Ropivacaine	2–4 h	fast	

Fig. A5.1

Fig. A5.2

Fig. A5.3

Fig. A5.4

Abram SE. Volume VI: Pain management. In: Miller RD (ed.), Atlas of anesthesia. Edinburgh: Churchill Livingstone, 1992.

Abram SE, Haddox D. The pain clinic manual, 2nd edn. Philadelphia, PA: Lippincott Williams and Wilkins, 2000.

Benumof JL. Clinical procedures in anesthesia and intensive care. Philadelphia, PA: Lippincott Williams and Wilkins, 1991.

Brown DL. Atlas of regional anesthesia, 2nd edn. Philadelphia, PA: WB Saunders, 1999.

Cousins MJ, Bridenbaugh PO (eds). Neural blockade in clinical anesthesia and management of pain, 3rd edn. Philadelphia, PA: Lippincott -Raven, 1996.

Patt RB. Cancer pain. Philadelphia, PA: Lippincott-Raven, 1992.

Raj, P (ed.). Clinical practice of regional anesthesia. Edinburgh: Churchill Livingstone, 1991.

Wall PD, Melzack R (eds). Textbook of pain, 4th edn. Edinburgh: Churchill Livingstone, 1999.

Wildsmith JAW, Armitage EN (eds). Principles and practice of regional anaesthesia. Edinburgh: Churchill Livingstone, 1987.

INDEX